The
Feminine Fertility Cure

Discover Your Innate Power to Have a Baby
Regardless of Age, Diagnosis, or Scary
Statistics

ROSANNE AUSTIN

Published 2024

ISBN 979-8-9873031-3-9 (paperback)

ISBN 979-8-9873031-4-6 (eBook)

Proofread by Andrae Smith Jr., Lantern Literary

CONTENTS

For every woman who truly desires to live the life of her wildest dreams...and is committed to making those dreams her reality.

Want a FREE e-journal to help you awaken YOUR Fearless Feminine?

I have created journal prompts based on Feminine First Principles that will help you tap into your fertility super power —*the Fearless Feminine.*

As a big thank you for including this book in your fertility journey, I want to give you something special to capture your breakthrough moments with Fearless Feminine awesomeness! **No need to try to figure out your new feminine flow solo— I've got you, boo.**

Mindset is half the battle when it comes to fertility success, so let me help you tap into what makes you fearless, feminine, and FERTILE.

Get your *free* Feminine Fertility Cure e-journal NOW!

Scan the QR code or go to https://www.frommaybetobaby.com/ ffc-gift-1.

Chapter 1

The Real Problem with Your Fertility Isn't Your Diagnosis

I f this book is in your hands, there's at least one thing I know about you that other people might not. They don't know this about you because you don't want their pity, and you know they'd never *really* understand. You've shed tears over it at random times and in wildly inconvenient places. It's kept you up at night, scouring the far reaches of the internet for anything that smacks of a solution. It's caused you to second-guess just about every decision you've made in your adult life and even question your value as a woman. You, Mama, are struggling with fertility.

No matter what you've tried, you haven't been able to get and stay pregnant. The pain and shame have ripped your heart to shreds. There are moments when you feel okay, but that's only because you're temporarily distracted by something else (probably work or some BS you said yes to just to be "nice"), or you've thoroughly numbed with Netflix. Too often, when you are in earshot of someone innocently uttering a word about pregnancy or babies (funny how our hearing becomes wildly attuned to the slightest mention of anything proximately related to fertility!), the questions thundering around that beautiful head of yours are *Will my day ever come? Will I have my baby?*

You have tried every treatment, diet, lotion, and potion you can get your hands on. You've driven thousands of miles, searching for answers. You know more about your menstrual cycle than most reasonable women would. You've been poked and prodded. You've gotten your husband or partner to do and eat things that had him seriously questioning your sanity. Mama, you are in good company. There are millions of women who have trod this path, but with this book in your hands, you've come to a fork in the road that could put you on a path to fertility success you hadn't quite imagined. In fact, I'm willing to bet that the ideas in this book will cause you to take at least one bold new action that you'll later credit as the pivot point that finally put you on the path to baby-making success. Buckle. Up.

That said, let's start with an inquiry into an aspect of your fertility journey that I bet no one has had the guts or awareness to present.

What if the biggest problem with your fertility was set in motion before you were born and has nothing to do with dysfunction in your body? What if the real "problem" has been so insidiously hidden in plain sight that you wouldn't even notice it unless or until you began struggling with fertility? Even worse, what if it continues to silently undermine your heroic efforts to conceive until you start asking the dangerous questions that brought you to this book?

I'm doing "all the things," but nothing's working; what am I missing?

They can't tell me exactly what's wrong—is it ME?

I'm willing to do anything; will someone help me?

If you're asking questions like these, I'm willing to bet that you have the problem that I'm dragging out of the shadows and into the light with this book.

I Help Women Unf*ck This Problem Every Day

You're probably wondering how I can be so sure. I know you have this problem because I have spent the past ten years of my professional life coaching women from around the world to fertility success. I've gotten to know thousands of women living with this problem. These women were floored that they had it, and solving it not only changed their lives but was the primary catalyst for helping them get and stay pregnant when the cards were stacked against them. And when I say "stacked against them," I don't just mean a *little* stacked against them. I'm talking about women who were told they had a less than 1% chance of conceiving by any means. Women who had undergone state-of-the-art treatments for years with no success, who went on to get pregnant within months of implementing what I teach. These are women from ages twenty-eight to fifty-three, from the United States to Kenya, Singapore to Canada, and everywhere else in between. The efficacy of my work, my reputation as a loving straight-talker, and my experience of having spent seven years on this journey myself have made me the coach that even doctors turn to when they struggle to conceive.

I'm not sharing this from a place of hubris. Not even close. I'm sharing this because it's what I know to be true. I know you might be skeptical. I know that if someone were about to tell me what I am going to tell you, I would have probably shaken my head—*at least at first*. I was a prosecutor in California when I lived my own fertility journey. I was the most suspicious and skeptical person you could possibly meet. It was my job to be that way. But when I realized I had been scammed, I couldn't unsee it. When I started addressing the real problem with my fertility, my husband and I did something we were basically told was impossible: we conceived and had our son Asher naturally, when I was almost 44, after years of treatment failure. This is how powerful what I am sharing in this book is.

I don't care how long you've been trying to conceive, what your diagnosis is, what percent chance of success you've been given, or how many times you've failed on this journey. When you dare to ask the questions I will ask and explore the ideas I will share, you can turn things around. My clients and I are living proof.

Mama, You've Been Scammed

Well, let me be clear: it's not just you. As I said earlier, I was scammed too. In fact, generations of American women have fallen prey to the scam.

What's the scam I'm talking about? Simply put, we were led to believe that our feminine nature is incompatible with "real" success. This misdirection has led to a systematic masculinization of women in this country. This reality has had a measurably devastating impact on our fertility and, ultimately, our quality of life. Said another way, we've been taught to behave like men, and we are paying for it dearly with our fertility. We see proof of this both socially and biologically. In fact, this scam has helped create nothing short of a fertility emergency in the United States. Our plummeting birth rate and skyrocketing infertility rates prove it.

Wait, what, Rosanne? I wear makeup, own a few dresses, have been known to wear super cute heels, and watch the occasional Hallmark movie! How am I acting like a man, and how can that possibly be messing with my fertility?

I promise I will explain this more in the coming chapters, but to give you a sense of what we are dealing with, women have been conned into subordinating our innate feminine desire for love, babies, family, and meaningful community to a masculine paradigm of "success" that invariably lies outside of the home and treats the longing in our hearts as if it were provincial prudishness. We were sold the idea that to "get ahead," we had to adopt more masculine traits and suppress our femininity. We have been propagandized into believing that motherhood is the lesser choice and that if we choose to exercise that choice, it's only reasonable *after* we have checked the boxes of masculine success first—higher education, consistent career advances, and the amorphous state of "financial stability." By the time we get "there," all too often, we have found ourselves in a position where our fertility is at best diminished and at worst in peril.

What's so cleverly insidious about the scam is that it's couched as "progress." Doubt this? Ask yourself, *How often were you actively and enthusiastically encouraged as a little girl to consider staying home, having babies, and nurturing a family as a viable and responsible option for your life?* Unless you were raised in very specific communities, chances are, your answer to that question is *never* or was limited to an isolated conversation you had with an older relative, whose wisdom you blew off as antiquated nonsense or the dawdling dalliances of dementia. Seriously, when was the last time you heard about a relative or acquaintance who chose to start her family in her early twenties before pursuing higher education or a career, and you genuinely thought to yourself, *Good for her*? I bet if presented with those facts, you'd have more questions than congratulations.

The reality is that most of us were raised with the steady anthem of " 'smart' girls go to college," "make your own money so you don't have to 'depend' on a man," "wait to have a family until you are 'established' in your career" (whatever that means), and a host of other one-sided garbage that has led scores of American women to hit their mid to late thirties and early forties childless and scrambling in a panic to have babies when they realize their lives are empty, disconnected, and, if we are brutally honest, horribly unsatisfying. We were basically taught that there was only one "successful" way to live—and that wasn't a way led by feminine pursuits.

Think back to when people asked about your plans after high school. I bet you didn't spend any time talking about getting married, having babies, and raising a family. Your answer was likely about where you were accepted for college or what profession you planned to pursue. If someone pressed further and asked about your plans for a family, you probably would've responded (slightly irritated or embarrassed) with something vague like "maybe someday." If you are anything like me, it would have felt weird and even offensive to suggest that you choose something other than an education and career.

I'm sure that there's one woman you remember from school who opted to get married and focus on her family, and you probably thought to yourself, *Poor thing threw her life away...She had so much potential!* That's not because you are a judgmental jerk. It's because that's the message we've been fed for decades—home, family, and traditionally feminine pursuits are the lesser choices. This same *lesser choice* judgment comes up when a woman does something "radical" like decide to stay home and not go back to work after her maternity leave. You can already hear the scuttlebutt around the watercooler being something to the effect of, "*Tsk, tsk, what a shame. She had such a promising career!*" You know this is true, and chances are that you've probably thought some of these things yourself. And that only proves my point. Ask yourself, though: if having babies and families is the lesser choice, why are so many educated, high-achieving women desperate to do it? Because it's *not* the lesser choice. It's awesome, and deep down on some level, if we are honest, it's what we've wanted all along.

Your Struggle with Fertility Is a Wake-Up Call—Go with It

I realize that all this talk about women taking on more masculine traits and family being the "lesser" choice may have your head spinning. You may be questioning why you picked this book up in the first place. You might be confused by what I mean when I say *femininity*. Don't worry; we'll get there. Leveraging your femininity will become the fertility superpower you had no idea you needed. Just know that any pushback you might have to what I'm raising here is *exactly why you need to keep reading.*

As human beings, it's our nature to resist anything that challenges our deeply held worldviews. Any pushback or resistance you feel coming up is clear evidence of the masculine paradigm operating in your life. The last thing it wants is to lose its cushy-cozy spot in your mind. Beware! The masculine paradigm loves to use weapons like frustration, anger, offense, mockery, rejection, and blame in defense of its hegemony. If you feel any of those things...great! It means you are in the masculine matrix, but that bugger is starting to squirm. That's exactly what we want.

As I will explain, when you are trying to conceive, living by a masculine paradigm is not only miserable, but it can block your baby. You needn't look further than your own fertility journey to see proof. The fear, doubt, negativity, shame, guilt, overwhelm, and exhaustion you feel? Those are undeniable evidence of the masculine paradigm at work. The good news is that I have helped otherwise highly educated, super-successful women who didn't have a clue that being disconnected from their femininity could negatively impact their fertility reclaim it. And, when they did, they quickly got on track to fertility success.

I also know that, on some level, the idea that what has made you successful in your professional life could be negatively impacting your fertility success may conjure up some mixed feelings. That's okay. Rest assured that none of what I'm sharing here is about blaming you for choices you've made in the past. I suspect you're already pretty good at that and don't need my help, and even if you did, I wouldn't be an accomplice to such abuse. I see the fertility journey as a wake-up call, a check engine light of sorts that's telling us that something isn't working properly. I want you to be a raging fertility success. That is why, in this book, we are exploring a topic that most ignore, discount, or even laugh at: *how a reclamation of your femininity will be a key component to your fertility success.*

I'm willing to bet that you've done far weirder sh*t in the name of conceiving this baby than rediscovering your femininity, so go with it, sister. This may be the most fun you've had on this journey.

Your Instincts Are Right: You Are Trying to Get Pregnant Like a Man

I am certain that some part of you has suspected that your way of life and your pursuit of success have had something to do with your struggle with fertility, even if you hadn't quite characterized either of those things as "masculine" in nature. Sometimes women beat themselves up over wanting too much, being "too career-focused," or "waiting too long" and tend to treat those realities as individual character flaws rather than as the consequence of social, familial, or cultural conditioning. As I will share later in this book, for decades, women have been taught to embrace masculinity to such a degree that we lose connection to our femininity. That loss of connection becomes wildly apparent when we try to do inherently feminine things with a masculine approach. This brings us to a topic near and dear to my heart: *trying to get pregnant like a man.*

I must admit, saying the phrase *trying to get pregnant like a man* makes me chuckle, not only because it's ludicrous, but because it's a frighteningly accurate description of the insanity I see women trapped in. *Trying to get pregnant like a man* describes the state where women are so consumed with conception that they apply masculine principles of achievement, working harder, competition, comparison, scarcity, pushing past pain, forcing, perfectionism, and an arbitrary timeline to their fertility journey. I've seen this play out in countless ways, but some of the most common are women agonizing over their fertile window to the point where they go into a tailspin if their husband or partner isn't game for sex at the exact second that window opens, having back-to-back IVF cycles to the point of exhaustion because they are afraid time is running out, or steering almost every personal conversation into one about conceiving. Trying to conceive quickly goes from being a celebration of love, approached with excitement, joy, and ease, to something a woman must chase, earn, and suffer for. Often, it isn't until I point out the fact that she's *trying to get pregnant like a man* that a woman even stops to consider the fact that she might be trying to do the most feminine thing she can possibly do as a woman...*like a man*! She is so stuck in "Man Mode" (which I will explain further in the next chapter) that she doesn't know how to get out.

Every single woman I have had the good fortune of pointing this out to has looked back at me wide-eyed as if to say, in an old-timey voice, "Great Scott, you're right!" We instinctively know there's something "wrong" with this approach, even if, up till now, we didn't have the language for it and didn't know what to do about it.

While it's true that you might have some polysyllabic diagnosis that super smart doctors have told you is impacting your fertility, from my experience in the trenches, having coached thousands of women to fertility success despite those "scary" diagnoses, the real solution to your fertility issues isn't found solely in addressing any physical or biological issues. You and your body are far more complex than that. If you've been on your fertility journey long enough, you know that if the solution were as simple as a diet, pill, or treatment, we'd all do those things and never struggle a day on this journey again. If you've ever been told your uterine lining was "perfect," your hormone levels were "great," and everything "looked good," yet failed to get pregnant, you know exactly what I mean. This is why I know the most effective fertility cure must include an improved connection to the feminine—and when I share the details and data, you will understand exactly why.

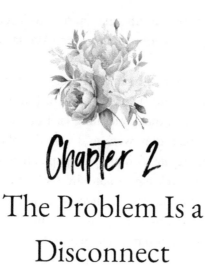

Chapter 2

The Problem Is a
Disconnect

Before we dive into detail on this masculine versus feminine thing and why it's messing with your fertility, let's zero in on something extremely important to keep in mind as we move forward. As I said in chapter 1, your struggle with fertility is a wake-up call. That's not meant as a cutesy little quip to create a false sense of urgency or importance; it's a fact. The feminine within you has been trying to get your attention for a while. She's tried exhaustion (which you've plowed through) and glimpses of intuition (which you often ignore); she's told you when your relationships suck (yet you stay too long), and she's told you to say a bold no (but you stick to your people-pleasing yes). The reason you can't afford to ignore her call now is that fertility is inherently feminine. *You need her.* Your results to this point show you just how badly you need her. Getting and staying pregnant is solely in the realm of the feminine. If you are at all serious about succeeding on this journey, you can't ignore her any longer. She's your fecundity BFF. Just think, if all the masculine, fear-based fighting, controlling, forcing, competing, and self-flagellation you've been engaging in was going to get you to Mama Town, you'd be there by now.

There are millions of women in this country (one in five at the time of this writing[1]) struggling with fertility and walking around with a sense that something isn't quite right. They are doing all the things they were told would make them happy, but the truth is, they *aren't* happy. On paper, they should be, but they aren't. They can't figure out why. On top of that, they are doing all the things people tell them to do to get and stay pregnant, but none of those things are working. They have spent decades listening to what other people have told them to do while completely disconnected from where the answers actually lie.

A Call Back to the Feminine Is a Gift

Brace yourself. I am about to say something that may completely change the way you look at your fertility journey.

Without the *gift* of a struggle with fertility and the inkling of awareness that caused you to pick up this book, you aren't likely to have discovered what's *really* going on in your life. That's not because you're an idiot; it's because the disconnection with your feminine has been conditioned out of you so deviously that you couldn't see the sleight of hand, and you were so anesthetized to the pain of her excision with "progress" that it isn't until you *need* her that the pain of her absence can be felt. Fertility is so inextricably connected to the feminine that her message to you can't possibly be made more clear. Not only is she standing in front of you waving a red flag, but she's

---

1. "Infertility FAQs," Centers for Disease Control and Prevention, last updated April 26, 2023, https://www.cdc.gov/reproductive-health/infertility-faq/index. html.

backed by a high school marching band playing a valiant rendition of Aretha Franklin's "Respect." Your feminine has been trying to get your attention, and your fertility is her messenger. Be glad for this because your feminine isn't just going to give you a baby; she's going to give you your life back.

A struggle with fertility forces us to confront our relationship with our feminine. Wise women will see that. Mother Nature operates on a mercilessly strict principle of *f*ck around and find out*. When you starve your feminine for long enough, there is a price to pay. Consider yourself lucky that you're becoming aware of this now, not later, *when it could be too late*. Women who haven't lived this journey and, therefore, aren't forced to look at their relationship with femininity in such a direct way are likely to blow off the feeling of unsettled unhappiness, attributing it to being hormonal, wanting too much, or simply needing to up the dosage of their antidepressants and get on with their lives. They'll take a two-by-four to the face from old Mama Nature in some other way. Not that I'd wish that on anyone, but it's simply a fact. Mother Nature's cadre of resources is deep and diverse. She might use overwhelm, self-sabotage, creative impulse, spiritual awakening, overeating, career change, nonfertility health crises, and a litany of other measures to get the attention she desires. In either case, the more you ignore her, the higher she will ratchet up her communications, and the less you will like the results.

When you're trying to get and stay pregnant, you don't have the luxury of blowing off a call from your feminine. Take heed. Here's why.

Fertility Issues Reveal Wounds to the Feminine

Getting pregnant and giving birth to your baby is the most feminine experience you can possibly have. I am repeating this intentionally—because if you are disconnected from your feminine, you can't hear it enough. You are bringing forth life!

As women, our bodies give us this incredibly unique life-giving power. When our body isn't working the way we expect, it strikes a blow to the core of who we believe we are. Fertility issues trash how we see ourselves as women because our ability to have a baby is usually taken as a given. When that *given isn't giving*, you start questioning things you might not have otherwise questioned.

A struggle with fertility isn't just a series of bad days. It's not vague or generalized unhappiness. It's an existential crisis that doesn't go away with the promise of a vacation, new car, or new job. It's driven by a heart-based primal longing. The pain of not having that need fulfilled doesn't go away. Over time, it may become a dull ache, but there isn't a day that goes by when you aren't reminded of it. Women in the thick of it start using language like "less of a woman" or "broken," which speaks not only to the obvious biological aspects of fertility, but, I believe, indicates burgeoning awareness of the deeper, more profound disconnect with their femininity. I stand firm with my characterization of the disconnect with femininity as more profound in its implications than a biological or physical issue because a woman's connection to her femininity will determine how she resolves those issues. There's no pill or treatment alone that can help a woman get and stay pregnant if she is either consciously or unconsciously rejecting the wants, needs, desires, and expression of her feminine. The fertility journey is a feminine problem bringing your attention to a problem with your femininity. This is true even if your partner is the one with a fertility issue—because the whole truth is that you both play a role.

Further proving my point, the need to label and directly or indirectly blame is a masculine defense mechanism. It's a huge indicator that your feminine *is* out of whack and you are living your fertility journey in Man Mode.

Doubt that? Keep reading.

Man Mode Explained

If you are wondering whether you are currently living your fertility journey in Man Mode or actively *trying to get pregnant like a man*, let's peruse some of the telltale signs, shall we?

- You've told yourself at least a thousand times that if you just *worked harder* and were *more "perfect,"* your baby would get here.
- You torture yourself for waiting so long, being too old, and wanting so much.
- You've repeatedly felt like screaming, "Will someone just tell me what to do? I will do it! I will do *anything!*"
- You compulsively compare yourself with pregnant women you see, wondering what's wrong with *you.*
- Your daily fertility routine has multiple steps and includes a ghastly number of supplements and gadgets, and you are constantly worried you aren't *doing it "right."*
- You scrutinize your partner's compliance with the Frankensteined fertility "program" you've cooked up for them based on what you've read online and bits of what your fertility team has shared, and if they waver in the least bit, you nag at them for not being committed to this baby.
- Your personal and professional calendars are dominated by notes about when your next fertile window or treatment cycle ends or begins, and fertility appointments take precedence over any other events.

- You beat yourself up for your level of investment in treatments, supplements, and coaching, to such a degree that you feel shame and use phrases like "I've done all these things, and I'm still empty-handed."
- There is a sinking feeling in your stomach that you're running out of time, that things aren't happening fast enough, and that if this baby doesn't "happen" soon, it ain't happening.
- You struggle to tell your partner, friends, family, and coworkers what you really want—and you fear what might happen if they find out!
- At times, you feel so exhausted and burned out by this journey that you wonder if you really want this baby after all, and you toy with giving up.

Whether you identify with one or all these signs, whether you feel them once a week or on the hour, what we are talking about here is your thoughts and behavior being dominated by masculine energy. These signs show that you are a woman who is thinking—and therefore operating—by masculine measures and expectations, which is the essence of Man Mode. You can feel the grinding nature of it. It's about approaching this journey from a perspective of working, earning, getting, competition, lack, scarcity, and fear. At the core of that approach is the belief that you aren't enough. It's all about the hunt, the chase, and *proving you can do it*, which, even if you are new to this masculine versus feminine stuff, is so patently masculine. When I refer to *trying to get pregnant like a man*, this is exactly what I am talking about.

I know part of you might argue that the behaviors I listed just show your "commitment" or are signs of how important having this baby is to you—in other words, they show you're "doing everything you can." But this argument, which assumes the masculine way is the only way to succeed, just proves my point. Who says you must work harder or be more "perfect"? What has competition with others or relentlessly beating yourself up done to improve your fertility? Who says there's a "right way" to do this journey? How will punishing yourself with a crushing, hectic fertility lifestyle put a baby in your arms? Where in all of this craziness are *you*, as your own unique woman, taken into consideration?

If you're reading this book, living your journey in Man Mode hasn't worked. It's woefully out of alignment and can continue to create disastrous results. You, your baby, your partner, and your well-being deserve better.

Let's talk more about this masculine and feminine thing in detail so you'll be able to identify it and stop letting it sabotage your fertility.

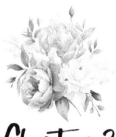

Chapter 3

Understanding the
Masculine and Feminine

Whether you already knew all about the masculine and feminine or had ever used those terms before starting this book, I'm willing to bet you understand instinctively that it doesn't make sense to try to do such an intensely feminine thing as conceiving from Man Mode. You may not know exactly why this is yet, but we will get there.

Now, if you have the problem I'm describing in this book, I probably have some *'splaining* to do to help you understand. Let's start with some basics, and then I will get more specific about what I mean by masculine and feminine energy.

We all have masculine and feminine energy within us— regardless of whether we are male or female. These energies have nothing to do with gender roles; rather, they have to do with the distinct energy we bring to what we do, how we behave, and the way we think. The masculine and feminine within us work cooperatively and are not necessarily opposites. I like to think of them as groupings of characteristics that make up who we are, and while they may be expressed to varying degrees in each person, they are nonetheless expressed in everyone.

We are designed to maneuver between our masculine and feminine throughout the day so that we can respond to situations and needs that show up in our lives from moment to moment. I'm not alone in believing it's part of the divine design for us to have these sides of ourselves, as we see the concept of the yin (feminine) and yang (masculine) come up as far back as at least the third century BCE in China.[1] One example of our ability to move between the masculine and feminine situationally, throughout the day, would be the vigilant energy we take on when participating in a serious, possibly contentious, meeting at work (masculine) versus the compassionate energy we bring to a coworker who is crying because her mom passed away (feminine.) Instinctively, you can see the difference between these energies. Certainly, the masculine and feminine can be more subtle than the examples given, but we'll get there.

No Right or Wrong, but There Is an Ideal

It's important to note here that, by pointing out the differences between the masculine and the feminine, I'm not saying that one is good, bad, weak, or strong. The masculine and feminine both have their merit, utility, time, and place. I don't believe we can function to the best of our ability without leaning in to the distinct advantages of both. When we get stuck in one energy, we get into real trouble, and that is at the core of what I'm teaching you about in this book. I believe the ideal for all of us is to marshal the full range of these energies within us in a way that reflects our unique values and personality. Doing so not only allows us to cope with the ups and downs of our lives, but

---

1. "Yinyang," *Encyclopedia Britannica*, last modified December 4, 2023, https://www.britannica.com/topic/yinyang.

it gives us access to a level of internal resources we would not otherwise be aware of.

To be clear, I am not suggesting that anyone needs to make an extreme pendulum swing from being in their masculine to being in full feminine mode. Going to extremes is just more of the masculine paradigm at work. As we move forward, you will see that what I will teach you here is about finesse and finding the right mix for you. I will discuss that more, particularly within the context of femininity and fertility, later. For now, let's keep exploring what makes these energies unique.

Manifesting the Masculine

Masculine energy is referred to as *masculine* because it's based on the behaviors and traits of men. This unquestionably has its roots in biology, as we see masculine behavioral traits in men, regardless of culture. Masculine energy is associated with being the protector, hunter, doer, and thinker. It's the part of us that strives, chases, achieves, executes, works, overworks, and *crushes it*. The masculine is the foundation of much of our outward success. He cares less about cooperation and what others think than he does about victory at any cost. He's the part of us that keeps moving forward when we are tired or want to quit. He's all about sheer force of will and is likely to shout, *I'll rest when I'm dead!*

There is a seriousness and weightiness to masculine energy. He tends to be vigilant and defensive, as he anticipates worst-case scenarios and a constellation of what-ifs. This makes perfect sense, as he is, after all, the protector in us. This is also why the masculine tends to focus on lack, scarcity, and the preservation of resources, as opposed to the more feminine perspective of abundance. The masculine is also associated with the so-called *logical, level-headed* side of us, which is less concerned with heart-based choices and instead focuses on facts, figures, probabilities, and what is reasonable. The masculine makes decisions based on the current landscape and circumstances, rather than faith and intuition. Suffice it to say that the cost-benefit analysis made from the masculine is completely different from that made from the feminine.

Interestingly, while the masculine may seem serious and sober, he is also the part of us that seeks adventure and is less drawn to putting down roots.

When thinking about how you can tell if you are in your masculine, I have always said that the most consistent measure is when something *feels like work*. That's not necessarily a bad thing, but it is distinct from what I feel is being in the creative flow of the feminine. The work I'm talking about feels more like a grind of productivity, than losing yourself in a task because you love it so much. I know I'm in my masculine when I'm relying on discipline, determination, and grit. This doesn't just apply to *literal* work though. I have observed that one is in masculine energy when their relationships feel like work as well. It's when we just *suck it up* and don't say anything, for the sake of keeping the peace and just getting through something, rather than engaging in feminine expression of truth. It's true that there are countless other ways the masculine can manifest, but when it feels like you are pushing, controlling, running yourself to exhaustion, and just trying to "get through it," you are without a doubt manifesting your masculine.

The Fascinating Feminine

If you hazard that the feminine is associated with traits held by women, you're right on target. The feminine is the creative, intuitive, curious, sensual, spiritual, nurturing, and vulnerable side of you. She's the part of you that loves feeling beautiful, that's playful, receptive, and perceptive. The feminine loves to talk about her dreams, passions, and plans, whether or not she knows exactly how to get there or when. You can be certain that the masculine will demand those details from her at some point. The feminine is the part of you that knows exactly what to say to defuse a tense situation and remembers the details that make people feel special. It's this level of sensitivity that makes the feminine not only more emotional, but also more emotionally intelligent and intuitive. Feminine energy allows us to adeptly *read the room* and notice subtlety that the masculine would clumsily bulldoze over. The feminine is also less concerned with sticking to a predictable plan than she is with how a process feels, allowing her to adjust on the fly. The feminine is all about heart-based creative expression and following one's passion. Decisions made from the feminine have more to do with positive possibilities than they do with pessimistic probability. They are decisions made from faith, regardless of current circumstances, and often seem risky to those who don't share a vision fueled by the feminine.

The feminine craves a sense of groundedness and home. In addition to this sense of home, the feminine desires a level of security, predictability, and protection to feel safe. While the feminine desires safety, there is an undeniable optimism that is inherent to her. I believe this is connected to the deeply spiritual nature of the feminine. In fact, that spirituality and connectedness to something higher is one of the most consistent qualities I've observed in those I've met who exude authentic feminine energy. This speaks to the receptivity and openness that is inherently feminine. It's for this reason that I repeat to my clients—as I do here—that conceiving is all about receiving.

Ultimately, the feminine is the part of you that longs for this baby and knows with all of her heart that some way, somehow, this baby is coming.

Now, you're probably wondering, "How the hell can I tell if I am in my feminine?" First off, if you're asking that question, you are most definitely not in your feminine. I say that with love, because the feminine is all about feeling. When you are stuck in the masculine, you tend to go a bit numb. When you are in the realm of the feminine, your focus is from the neck down. My clients hear me excitedly shout *"neck down!"* when I want them to engage their feminine. When I say that, I'm telling them to get out of the myopic illusion of masculine logic. Thinking and logic aren't your only faculties. Nor are they the wisest to use in every situation. There's more to us than that. We have intuition and imagination, which are incredibly valuable and offer solutions that are not only exciting, they swing feminine! When your heart and senses are engaged, you are in the feminine. This is why there's a peace and softness to the feminine that's unmistakable. The feminine is inherently about ease. When you let things come to you, you're in the feminine. When you let go of the need to control and are instead focused on curiosity and noticing how you feel and the details around you, you're in the feminine. She's all things delicious and sensory. It's also when you are sensitive and tapped into your spiritual side that you are absolutely in your feminine. This connectedness, presence, and embracing of feelings is all feminine, all day! I also see resilience as deeply feminine, because for me, resilience is about being aware of the truth of our experiences, appreciating them for what they are, and using them to propel us forward. It's deeper and richer than just relying on grit and force. It's a persistence that demonstrates an understanding and perspective that powering through just doesn't have. Remember that when you are inclined to rely solely on your masculine to get by. And, in the end, when you allow yourself to drop the judgment and enjoy the moment, you are definitely in your fabulous feminine.

The Feminine Isn't a One-Trick Pony

As women, our feminine is at the core of who we are, regardless of how we uniquely express it. Every woman is different, and therefore, so is her feminine. I want to assure you that as you explore your feminine, it's not all about pink, sparkly sh*t and unicorns. Remember that the feminine is creative, she's sensual, and she's connected spiritually, so all that influences how she is expressed in our lives. In many ways, she's like a fingerprint. For some women, she will indeed be expressed in things like beautiful dresses, lace, makeup, and bouncy hair. But even in those traditional outward expressions, she will unquestionably have some twists. She can show up in less obvious ways, such as a unique cadence of speech or silky blouse that Madame chose just because it felt good on her skin. Or she can show up in leather and combat boots, making her presence known through Madame's ease and grace as she walks into the room. To be clear, the feminine isn't only expressed through outward appearance; she can also be felt in someone's way of being. Some of the most feminine women I have had the good fortune of interacting with have had the outward trappings of the masculine, but the moment you are in their presence, you can just...*feel* it. Its ease, softness, gentle wisdom, and authentic engagement, to name a few things.

It's time we all let go of the feminine caricature of being "girly" and traded up for unique expression that's just feminine AF. Rather than overintellectualizing this, I would encourage you to lovingly woman-watch. Next time you are out and about, take a good look at the women around you and see if you can spot how they express their feminine. It's fascinating and inspiring. Your own feminine expression will be as unique as you allow her to be.

The Dark Side of the Extremes

Extremism of any kind is a solid indicator that something isn't right. Extremes and absolutes signal that discernment and subtlety have been thrown out the window, in favor of intellectual and emotional laziness and fear. Not a great way to live. I believe the same is true when it comes to how we manage our masculine and feminine.

By now, you have gotten the basic message that disconnection from your feminine and overreliance on your masculine are *no bueno*. I will get to exactly how that impacts your fertility (patience!), but I want to shed some light on the other extreme. Let's talk about the feminine gone wild.

To this point, I've described the upside of the feminine. But she does have a dark side. I like to call her *Parking Lot Girl*, or PLG for short. Parking Lot Girl is the chick in the Chili's parking lot at 1:00 a.m. with mascara dripping down her face, one shoe on, shouting that she can't find her keys. Hot. Mess. PLG is the version of the feminine that, frankly, all of us who are trying to recover from being deeply entrenched in our masculine are afraid of. We don't want to be her, we don't want to be around her, and we don't even want to think about her. She is the essence of extreme vulnerability and is so overly reliant on her scattered, at times explosive, emotion that she's repellant. PLG is all over the place in her life; she can't make a decision because she's constantly changing her mind based on her horoscope; she's needy; she rarely pays bills on time; she's all about ideas, but lacks the ability to execute. PLG rejects her masculine because she thinks he will fence her in, not realizing that her masculine, marshaled properly, is there to provide helpful discipline and structure. She talks about wanting a Prince Charming, but when he rolls up on his steed with her missing shoe and keys, she calls him *boring*. Her femininity is cringey, because in its extreme, it turns into flighty weakness that's just plain gross. Like the messes we create when we are dominated by our masculine, overreliance on the feminine has messiness in kind.

It's All About the Interplay

It bears reinforcement here that I am not arguing in favor of the masculine or feminine being superior, nor am I stating that the descriptions I have given here are by any means exhaustive. They are a starting point. I believe those definitions become more refined in our individual lives with time, as they have in mine. The point is to begin understanding these parts of ourselves so we can move between them in a way that's authentic to each of us. The interplay between the two is fascinating and a lot like a dance.

While we'll go into greater detail on what you can do to start living from your Feminine First (aka your Fearless Feminine) for fertility and a fabulous life in a later chapter, I want to give you some basic ideas about what that can look like. Feminine First is leading with your creative, curious, spiritual, intuitive, nurturing, sensual, and loving self, then allowing your masculine side to help you bring your desires to fruition. Your Fearless Feminine is your unique expression of femininity and is the result of living by Feminine First principles. When operating from a Feminine First perspective, you won't wake up and immediately scramble for your phone so you can start attacking the seven thousand emails you got overnight. Nope! Instead, you'll allow yourself to gently rise, thank GUS (God/Universe/Source) for giving you another day, and think about what your intention will be. As you move through your day at work, you'll check in with yourself about whether you need to start saying no to new projects or cases, instead of mindlessly saying yes to whatever gets tossed your way. You'll tell people the truth about what you desire—*and get it*, instead of settling for the scraps tossed your way because of your addiction to people-pleasing politesse.

Within these examples is the interplay between the masculine and the feminine. Were you able to spot it? Let's dissect the first example to be sure you are following along. Getting up and connecting with GUS is feminine. The discipline to resist picking up your phone and immediately diving into the emails is masculine. Stuck in your masculine, you would have pushed right past all the good GUS stuff and gone right into email panic, thus starting your day off with a big old steaming bowl of misery. *Ick!* In the second example, deciding whether it's time for a well-placed *no* is feminine. Continuing to say *yes* out of fear would be masculine. In the last example, knowing what your truth is would be feminine, telling it would be masculine, and the people-pleasing is your PLG feminine.

I bet you're starting to get this! It's exciting because it will help you see the power in what I will be sharing in the next chapter.

Goal-Oriented, High-Achieving Women Take Heed

While you are starting to see the value of the interplay between the masculine and feminine, the problem is that American women are stuck in one gear, and we are paying dearly for it—in large part with our fertility. Your fatigue, burnout, and current struggle prove it.

To my earlier point in chapter 2 about Man Mode, as goal-oriented, high-achieving women, we get trapped in a pattern of behavior and belief that keeps us stuck in our masculine energy. We keep doing, striving, giving, performing, saving, helping, proving, and fighting, and we forget how to do anything else. Man Mode gets us to the point where we are so disconnected from our feminine that we have no clue who or what she is. Then we wonder why we can't just snap our fingers and get pregnant.

I consciously spent time on the subject of defining the masculine and feminine, their common traits, and how they might look in your life for a reason. Most of us, regardless of our level of education, are ignorant to what they are and how they influence our lives. Even if you took a bunch of women's studies courses, I'm not sure that the masculine and feminine would have been broken down in the way I just did so—apolitical and focused on energy. I can't know for sure, because my masculine rolled my eyes at those classes and had me avoid them like the plague. *Tee-hee-hee!*

This leads me to ask a delightfully daring question. How did a couple generations of women become so uniformly disconnected from their feminine to the point where they basically reject her?

I believe American women have been led to this ignorance, distrust, and, at times, disdain for the feminine over time, and it's brought us to the brink of destruction. I know that may sound dramatic, but the data on women's happiness and fertility prove it. I will share more about that later, but let's talk about how this is currently showing up on your fertility journey and in the rest of your life.

Chapter 4

Modern Women Are Stuck AF...And I Was Too

I f you look back carefully at the telltale signs of Man Mode I listed in chapter 2, you can probably see that this pattern of thought and behaviors isn't limited to how you are behaving on your fertility journey. I'm willing to bet this is exactly how you live other aspects of your life as well. Your struggle with fertility has simply amplified those characteristics because this is *the one* part of your life you can't outwork or control. What does a woman disconnected from her feminine do in that case? She doubles down on Man Mode because it has made her successful in the past, but she has no idea it's only pushing her further away from her baby.

Being stuck in Man Mode is why you're tired, why achieving feels empty these days, why you struggle to connect with your partner, and why you just keep working harder yet see little improvement in your life and on this journey. "Failing" is not normal for you, so you do what you've been taught—*work harder*.

When we are stuck in our masculine, everything becomes a

battle, to the point where it's just exhausting and we want to give up. As women, we pay a heavy price for living like men, physically, emotionally, and mentally—which, no surprise, creates toxic stress that plays out in our fertility. There is a point where everything that makes you so outwardly successful begins to suffer—your work, relationships, creativity, health, and connection to the vision you once had for your life. If you doubt this, ask yourself, *when was the last time you spoke to a woman who wasn't overwhelmed and crispy around the edges?*

When you are in Man Mode, are you really giving yourself the best possible chance to be open, receptive, nurturing, and welcoming to the potential for new life? Instinctively, you know the answer to that question. It's also why so many people around you are telling you to "take it easy" or, most annoyingly, "relax." Certainly, there are women out there stuck in Man Mode who do conceive, but when you are in a serious struggle with fertility, do you really want to use them as a yardstick? Would you really want to take the position that you don't have to change a thing when your heart, mind, body, and results thus far are telling you otherwise? No shade on those women, but their disconnection from their femininity may simply not have manifested in their fertility. They might have gotten pregnant with no issue at all, and that simply represents normal variation in human biology and experience, but that doesn't invalidate the position I'm taking. I assure you, it's biting those women in the ass in other areas of their lives.

The Big Fat Lie About Femininity

American women were sold a big fat lie about what it means to be feminine. We were told that our feminine was weak, untrustworthy, flighty, unproductive, too emotional, and dangerous and that if we were *too* feminine, we wouldn't be taken seriously. Even worse, we may have been led to believe that our feminine was unsafe. The version of femininity most of us were sold was akin to our old friend PLG from the previous chapter.

I speak from experience because I was once distrusting of—and at times repelled by—my feminine too. Sure, I'd let her slip out in small ways with my gorgeous Manolo Blahniks, works-of-art Hermès scarves, sleek, beautifully coiffed hair, and tidy makeup, but most of the time, I kept her locked in place and well-behaved with exquisitely tailored suits as I strode into the courtroom with armored-up masculine energy. I promise you, other than the sense to make a few great wardrobe selections, my connection to my feminine was in tatters. I didn't want to be PLG. The problem is that I was so ignorant and fearful of the feminine that I couldn't see that PLG was an extreme of what one could only *questionably* call feminine. It made sense that I was thinking that way; I was stuck in the masculine tendency to think in extremes.

At the time, there was nothing about me that was open, particularly soft, or receptive. If someone said to me, "Rosanne, you might want to be more feminine," I would have hissed and told them to get the f*ck out of my way—I had crime to fight! Sounds like I just *oozed* femininity, right?

My feminine reference point was my mom, and as much as I love her, given all of her complicated and at times explosive emotions and her dependence on my dad, I didn't want to be anything like her. That might sound harsh, but I'm just being real here. I love her with all my heart, and she is a fantastic human being, but I didn't want her life—or at least, *my possibly warped perception of her life.* From as early as I could remember, in school and at home, I was getting the message that femininity and feminine pursuits were frivolous and I should strive for more. I don't recall ever getting a counterargument for the feminine or clear messaging that said that the emotional, intuitive, spiritual, sensual, or creative side of me was safe and good.

The goal was for me to do well in school, go to college, get an advanced degree, and never, ever, *ever* have to depend on a man. That's what "smart" girls did. And so that's what I did, and it's what I continued to do until my struggle with fertility slapped me in the face and had me questioning everything about my life and the way I was living it.

I used to think I was a lone wolf freak for wrestling with this problem of disconnection from my femininity and generalized confusion about it. But when I started coaching women around the world through their fertility journeys, I saw that I wasn't alone. Disconnection from the feminine is an epidemic. Perfectly wonderful, kind, generous, insanely intelligent women, at the top of their professional games, were—and are! —stuck in their masculine and struggling to conceive. The more in their masculine they were, the harder it was for them to conceive. Like me, my ladies had one gear, and that's *go*. We sang the common anthem of overwork, under-receive, gut-out-the-pain, never-let-them-see-you-sweat perfectionism. It made us all very successful and put lots of letters after our names, but it left us all struggling to have the one thing we didn't realize we wanted so badly until it seemed impossible: babies. *Eeek!*

I saw this happening with ridiculous consistency, to women all over the world, from all kinds of upbringings, belief systems, and personal lives. It felt like we had all been told the same heartbreaking lie. And today, knowing what I know now, after ten-plus years in the trenches, seeing the effects and connecting the dots, there's no question in my mind that that's exactly what happened. Physicians, lawyers, teachers, nurses, engineers, bankers, artists, and business owners—we bought that lie hook, line, and sinker. And we didn't even see it coming.

My Fertility Was My Rude Awakening, Which Is Why I Know It's Yours

There's an interesting decision you have to make when you wake up and become aware that a bunch of stuff that you were told was right and true is simply part of a narrative, a half-truth, or downright false. You either keep it to yourself because you feel embarrassed, duped, and possibly question your sanity, or you do the opposite and tell everyone about it.

Honestly, I'm unbelievably glad I kept my awakening to myself at the time. When I realized that most of what I had been taught about the feminine and what being a "successful woman" means was based on a manipulatively misogynist agenda, I was floored. I could see the evidence of that truth in almost every aspect of my life. Most painfully, I realized it had controlled my sense of self-worth and kept me chasing after an unattainable ideal for years, leaving me exhausted, insecure, and consistently abandoning the truth in my heart. Talk about a dark night of the soul! Yes, the lies led me down a path that made me "successful" on paper, there's no doubt about that, but the truth was that I was failing at the things that really made me happy, most notably my relationships and calling in my baby. *My fertility was my wake-up call.*

While the path to reconnecting with my feminine involved many culminating events, the one that rubbed my face in the bloody fact that neglecting her could cost me everything—including my baby—was the miscarriage I had after using the last of the embryos my husband and I had created. Graphic characterization, I know, but my intent here is not to be gratuitous. I was so locked in my masculine that it wasn't until the intensity of that moment that I could see my situation clearly. The physical pain, the blood-soaked clothes, the rush to the emergency room on Christmas Day, the heartbreak, and the *what now* that consumed my life in the wake of that day forced me to see things about myself that I hadn't seen to the same degree before or had simply buried. Spending days and nights in a dark room, hopped up on codeine, intermittently wailing with grief, with episodes of *Downton Abbey* playing in the background as my body passed the pregnancy, I had a lot of time to think...*and feel.* No prior event in my life had knocked me down to such a degree of physical and emotional devastation. We had no more embryos. We were out of options. It looked like we were at the end of our baby-making road.

I had been working on my mindset for some time when the miscarriage happened. I learned to think in a completely different way, which brought to me the place where I did finally get pregnant. Instead of handing my power to statistics and naysayers, I cultivated the belief that, if the desire in my heart to be a mom was there, a way would be shown. And that's exactly what happened. That same skill set helped me move through the pain and grief of the loss. I knew that this wasn't the end of the road for me. The other thing that emerged in that moment, though at the time I didn't have language for it and couldn't quite describe it, was the beginning of my reconnection with my feminine. It was through my continued personal development work, encouraged by my feminine, that I finally gained the language to share it with you today. *Thank you, Fearless Feminine!*

The miscarriage lifted the veil of the masculine matrix I was living in. I couldn't just muscle through, try harder, or push further. It was painful to get out of bed, and I barely had the energy, so all I could do was lie there, facing what I had been feeling for some time. I was exhausted, depleted, and worried that I had been wasting my life, and I wasn't even sure who I was. As a prosecutor, I always had another move. I always had another argument. Everything about me to that point had been about pushing, competing, people-pleasing, and keeping up appearances, and I had never really stopped to ask myself scary questions like "Hey, is this really what I want? Is this even right for me?" I just did what family, friends, professors, the media, and society told me would be "success" and would make me happy. (It wasn't that I couldn't think for myself. I just didn't know any other way.) As the woman lying in bed, face smashed against a tear-soaked pillow, losing her baby, the next move wasn't so clear. That lack of clarity allowed me to be open to the part of me I needed so badly: my feminine. She showed up right on time, but the truth is, she had always been there.

Unlike the masculine, who needs immediate answers, hates ambiguity, demands evidence, is on guard, and doesn't have time for the spiritual, my feminine revealed herself to me, and I immediately fell into the peace of not having to know my next move. I knew it was my feminine because the energy I felt in that moment was gentle and nurturing. I know that might sound strange, very *Close Encounters of the feminine Kind,* but it wasn't little gray women coming out of a spaceship or some otherworldly apparition showing up in my bedroom that saved my ass. It was a faintly familiar feeling coming from within me. Instead of ignoring her whispers as I normally would, I rolled with her. From my feminine energy and perspective, I could simply *linger and be in the question of what was next for me.* The masculine side of me would have had a list of new clinics to call, fertility articles to read, and additional options mapped out that I could execute immediately. My feminine gave me authority to say no to all of that.

The other interesting thing I noticed during that time was a deep encounter with GUS. The feminine is the pathway to our spirituality. It's what opens our hearts and makes us receptive. My feminine allowed me to be open to GUS in that dark moment, instead of rejecting or blaming it. I wanted to know that everything would be okay and that a way to my son would continue to be shown. I remember praying for that repeatedly, and I remember a moment when what I call "a knowing" resonated through my body:

The same power that brought this baby will bring you your son.

I know how that might sound from where you stand today, but it's true. I no longer felt lack or despair. Instead, I knew that my son Asher was coming. I didn't know how or when, but *I knew he was coming.* My masculine was telling me that there was no chance, but my feminine told me that the past didn't matter; my boy was coming.

It was like a switch had been flipped. Instead of feeling like I had no more options—with no embryos left and nothing more that medicine could offer me—I felt free. It felt like, for the first time, I was free to believe whatever I wanted about my fertility, regardless of the statistics, because those buggers had done nothing *for* me. They kept me fearful and powerless. Changing my mindset had brought me to the place where, despite the heartbreak of a miscarriage and even though I was over forty and had no embryos to work with, *I had never been more optimistic about my prospects for pregnancy.* Crazy, right? I realized a critical aspect of the optimism, clarity, and freedom that I felt came from tapping into my feminine when I was at my lowest. This made me wonder what was possible if I continued exploring and including my feminine in my own development process. What my feminine was beginning to show me was the possibility that I could live and feel differently, and *I f*cking loved it.*

I'm not going to pretend that opening up to my feminine was easy. It required faith and a level of ovaries-deep surrender that, at the time, I wasn't sure I was capable of. But I couldn't deny how much better I felt. At the same time, what my feminine was showing me was a bit unsettling. I could see that so many of the masculine patterns I had been living by, the same ones that were making me successful professionally, were making me miserable personally. I was so stuck in Man Mode that I couldn't see how living that way was not only making it hard for me to conceive but was also slowly destroying my life. I wanted a deeper connection to my husband, I wanted work that fed my soul, I wanted to get to know the side of me that could believe bigger than her circumstances, I wanted to stop chasing approval and trying to please people who didn't have the slightest clue about who I really was, and I was tired of making myself wrong for the big, bold life I desired. I was tired of living by the lie that the only successful way for me to live was like a man. My feminine had been there for me when I needed her, and I decided to trust what she had shown me.

It's from that place that I began dismantling the lie about the feminine in my life. Not surprisingly, it was my feminine that told me I had to teach women what I had learned. My masculine was scared sh*tless because I had never been in business before, and I worried that no one would believe that a former prosecutor would have anything of value to say about fertility. *See that? There's that masculine programming again.* I had nothing but a failed pregnancy and a bold belief that mindset was the missing piece of the fertility puzzle. With no baby, none of what I was about to do made any sense. But as I began sharing what I had learned and my clients were getting pregnant left and right, my work caught fire, and since then, the results my clients create *have become a phenomenon.*

Beyond my work, I slowly began exploring and reclaiming my feminine by looking around my life and questioning the things in it. I began whittling away the things that no longer served me, and I made a practice of checking in with myself about whether each thing I was about to do *felt right.* The fact that I even stopped to consider my feelings was a big move for me. Having been stuck in my masculine for decades, it took time for my feminine to fully thaw. I started paying closer attention to what I liked and didn't like. I started opening my field of vision regarding what was possible for me. I began reconsidering what success meant and how I might measure it on my terms.

Responsibility Required Me to Write This: Mindset + The Feminine Works

Reclaiming my feminine was a process, one that I'm still continuing to this day, but the most convincing evidence of its transformative impact on fertility is how it made me more fertile in my forties than I was in my thirties! Yes, when medicine had nothing left to offer and, according to "the statistics," I had a snowball's chance in hell of getting pregnant naturally, I did exactly that: I got and stayed pregnant naturally.

Want to know how I did it? I made the conscious decision to work diligently on my mindset and go ovaries deep with my feminine. I wanted to see how far this dynamic duo could take me. I wanted to see how living with a mindset focused on possibility, fueled by my feminine, could change my life. In the twelve months leading up to the time that we conceived Asher, I decided to lean into my feminine by saying a *giant yes* to anything that felt right to me, lit me up, and would propel me forward in my life, my business, my marriage, and my future motherhood. It didn't matter how bold or crazy it seemed; I was doing it! My masculine worries about money, time, and "the how" had kept me stifled for too long. I wanted to have a completely different experience. Remember, the feminine is curious, sensual, and full of faith. I wanted all of that. All of it! For so many years, I had lived my journey in fear, doubt, and negativity. My feminine craved more and better than that. I wanted peace, joy, passion, and excitement again. My husband immediately jumped on board, 100% ready to support me in anything I decided to do, because who the hell wouldn't be attracted and excited to get down with that kind of energy? *Take note, Mama—that kind of feminine energy is infectious.*

My feminine craved things I had starved her of during our fertility journey, so here are some examples of the huge yeses I said when I let her take the lead:

- My feminine is insatiably curious and loves learning, so my husband and I began attending fun classes and personal development seminars together. I'd book 'em and we took 'em! *We even walked on hot coals at one of them!*
- Our fertility journey had isolated us and, in my masculine, I am deeply introverted, so my feminine urged me to widen our circle of friends and acquaintances so we could meet new people and make exciting new connections—which is exactly what we did.
- My feminine led me to create improved personal and professional boundaries that brought me incredible peace and relief. I started saying yeses to things that felt good to me and some long overdue noes to things that didn't.
- My feminine longed to have her influence show up more in my work, so I was more creative, open with my spirituality, and shared more about her in my teachings. This felt like a huge heart-based risk for me...and my clients loved it.
- There are few things my feminine loves more than luxury travel, and after years of not traveling at all because all our attention was on treatments, we booked an insane European vacation where our mantra was "If we want it, it's *yes.*"
- And, perhaps the most importantly, I said a big *yes* to my belief that my boy was coming. Believing in him was 100% feminine. My masculine obsession with numbers and probabilities had to go, and go for

good. I made the choice that I wasn't going back to my old ways. *I knew my fertility would be found in my feminine.*

That all started in October 2015, and by October 2016, I was pregnant *naturally*, for the first time in my life. We had Asher in June 2017, when I was within months of my forty-fourth birthday, and he was born healthy and strong. What this means is I went from years of struggle and heartbreak to getting pregnant naturally in less than a year, leveraging the power of mindset fueled by the feminine. Living that year in my feminine proved that I didn't have to be in Man Mode to get what I desired most in my life, including a booming business, a blissful marriage, and yes, a beautiful baby. My feminine had brought me better results in one year, without a single treatment or pharmaceutical, than I had experienced in the six years prior. The feminine quite literally compresses the timeline to your baby. My ladies and I are proof.

As I was working on the feminine within me, like I said earlier, I was seeing the same issue of "stuck in the masculine" coming up for my clients. When I started incorporating the discovery, exploration, and reclamation of the feminine in my own work, based on the results I had created for myself, I saw my clients' results becoming more dramatic and pregnancies begin happening even more quickly than before. Women who had faced less than 10% odds, who hadn't had periods in months, who had been told they were menopausal, and for whom IVF hadn't worked were getting pregnant naturally. In the end, whether a woman was trying to conceive naturally or with treatment didn't matter. The results were insane and, more importantly, *consistent.* It didn't matter the woman's age, prior diagnosis, number of past failures, or how long she had been trying to conceive. When she started implementing what I taught, she made getting pregnant no longer an *if*, but a *when.*

By combining sound mindset principles with an empowered relationship to the feminine, I've been able to help women get pregnant when they were told that doing so was "impossible."

Because this disconnect from the feminine and the systematic masculinization of women (which I will break down in chapter 5, because it is indeed systematic) that I've observed in myself and others is so pervasive and consistent, I feel a responsibility to share it with you here. There's a point when staying silent is ridiculous. With birth rates in the United States cratering,[1] I want to give women who are willing to see the truth an advantage. Women who reject the idea of embracing their feminine are on their own. I believe that mindset is and always has been the missing piece when it comes to fertility, but an essential aspect of mindset that will make you fertile AF is your relationship with the feminine. It's this nuance of femininity that makes my Fearlessly Fertile Method so effective and unique. As part of my methodology, I help my ladies undo the cultural damage that's been done to their femininity so they can be fearless, feminine, and fertile. When they tap into their feminine, they find a *gestational gear* they didn't know they had!

With a coaching practice full of women from all over the world presenting the same telltale signs of what I now call Fractured Feminine Syndrome f*cking with their fertility, I couldn't stay quiet anymore. But before we go there, let's talk more about exactly why femininity is so important and how being estranged from it can directly impact your chances of getting and staying pregnant. When you read what I have to say next, you'll want to get out of Man Mode pronto!

---

1. Melissa Kearney, Phillip Levine, and Luke Pardue, "The Mystery of the Declining U.S. Birth Rate," EconoFact, February 15, 2022, https://econofact.org/the-mystery-of-the-declining-u-s-birth-rate.

UNF*CK YOUR BELIEF ABOUT THE FEMININE—YOUR FERTILITY WILL THANK YOU

There may be part of you asking, "Well, what's so great about femininity? She sounds elusive, complicated, unsettling, and unfamiliar, and I might have to interrupt my already busy schedule to meet this Breezy B." Well, while she may be some of those things, at the same time, she's *none of those things*.

When we are exploring a topic that at times feels foreign, it helps to be reminded of what we are talking about. The feminine is the creative, intuitive, curious, sensual, spiritual, nurturing, and vulnerable parts of you. She's your whimsical playfulness, receptivity, and sensitivity. She's basically the opposite of the way you live your life now. When you are stuck AF in your masculine, you don't have ready access to these valuable qualities she offers. We can see how that's impacting you when we look at how living your fertility journey feels right now. Yes, *feels*. We are talking about the feminine, so let's feel some sh*t.

Living your fertility journey in the masculine feels like pushing, pulling, chasing, doubting, lacking, and never measuring up. The masculine is indeed the doer, the creator of structure. He gives you consistency and the grit-based ability to keep going. But, at the same time, he will drive you straight into a brick wall. He's an aspect of what makes you so strong, but being trapped in your masculine will drain you to such a degree that you go weak.

The feminine is a different kind of strength and empowerment. She's not better or worse; she's just different. The feminine gives you access to a constellation of faculties that, from a strategic standpoint, are well suited for the fertility journey. *How different would a day on your fertility journey feel if you were tapped into your creative, intuitive, sensitive, and spiritual?* You can't tell me that it wouldn't hit differently. Instead of the masculine keeping you running around like a chicken with your head cut off, desperately scrounging for solutions, your feminine would saunter in and get curious and creative. She'd ask questions like, "What's the solution that's here, but that I just can't see at the moment?" *OMG, seriously?* Tell me you can feel the difference between the masculine and feminine in that question alone!

The feminine is less about *doing* than she is about *being.* The feminine causes us to slow down to see, feel, and consider things the masculine will usher us past. The feminine is what tells you when a fertility clinic doesn't feel like a fit. She tells you when you need rest. She encourages you to meditate and pray. The feminine shows you where boundaries need to be set, while the masculine enforces those boundaries. The feminine is your connection to the intuition that whispers—or sometimes shouts—*"I know it doesn't look like it, but your baby is coming."* It's through our feminine that we meet our babies in our dreams and feel their presence so strongly in our visualizations that we shed tears. The feminine shows us truth that the masculine has no clue what to do with. *The feminine gives us access to information, inspiration, and resilience that, through the masculine alone, we can't reach.*

Speaking of resilience, let's talk about it for a moment. I mentioned this back in chapter 3, but it was only in passing. It warrants more attention here because it is so deeply connected to the feminine. *Who doesn't need resilience on this journey?* I see resilience as something completely different from your run-of-the-mill masculine stick-with-it-ness. It's informed by something much bigger than "just keep going." Resilience implies more than just mechanically moving forward. It's about drawing upon all of who you are, your experiences, and the vision you have for something better, which keeps you coming back, battle scars and all. It's more than simple *fight*. For these reasons, I see resilience as inherently feminine. When we are talking about something as unpredictable, heart-based, and demanding as the fertility journey, it's all about resilience. A successful fertility journey demands resilience and thereby requires the feminine.

The feminine has strength and information that is uniquely her own. She isn't all about the fall apart, as we have been led to believe. The uninformed love to blow her off as "crazy," but the truth is, she's crazy like a fox. Knowing what I know now, I can see that our old friend PLG is the crash you have when your feminine is in famine. (She needs the interplay with the masculine to feel fed.) The feminine we are talking about here is like the level-headed older sister, who intuits something isn't right for PLG, has the emotional maturity to call for a time-out, helps her find her keys, gives her a desperately needed hug, drives her home, and puts her to bed without judgment. The feminine knows she's valuable, can hold space for others, and plays by her own rules. The feminine is freaking awesome!

That's Great, Rosanne, But What's in It for My Fertility?

I know you want me to get to the part about how the disconnection from your feminine can f*ck with your fertility, so let's do that now. Your connection to your feminine, or lack thereof, is directly shaping three key components of success or failure on this journey: the mental, physical, and spiritual.

The mental piece of this equation comes down to the nature and quality of your decisions. The decisions you make are 100% the result of what you think and believe, aka your mindset. You might have heard me say this on my podcast or in my other books, but Thoughts → Beliefs → Actions → Results. It's logical, linear, and true. There is a dramatic difference in the nature and quality of decisions made from the feminine versus the masculine. I will unpack that.

When we make decisions solely from the masculine, we are looking at a set of facts in a very specific way. It's about numbers, statistics, "evidence," the past, judgment, what the "experts" or "authorities" say, price, timeline, and very concrete, tangible things. The posture of that decision, based on the description I have given, is defensive. Its focus is outward, largely centered on past events, and laden with limits. There is an undercurrent of fear, doubt, suspicion, and wanting to *see before one believes*. It's wildly risk-averse. Put another way, it's what some may describe as left-brain thinking.

There is obvious utility in decisions made from masculine energy. For the most part, we are taught to use the masculine in our decision-making because it appears to be more "logical" and not distracted by pesky emotions. Decisions from the masculine have a distinct quality about them, so let me give you an example so you can see how this plays out.

Let's say you're forty-one years old, and you've been on your fertility journey for four years. Other than struggling with fertility, you are reasonably healthy. You've tried a few different treatment interventions. You've changed your diet. You've done acupuncture. Your partner has been checked out, and all looks "good." Your doctor has run out of answers but tosses you the zinger that you have a less than 15% chance of getting pregnant.

You've thought about coaching with me, but you are scared it might not work for you—despite all the women you've heard on my podcast talking about how powerful and effective this work is. Your friends all have babies, your family is wondering how long you are going to "keep this up," and you've invested $75k in trying to conceive. *What would the masculine do with this set of facts?*

Everyone's masculine will certainly express differently, but having recovered from an overly dominant masculine myself and helped women around the world break free from their own traps, I'm going to give you my opinion on the kinds of thoughts and decisions the masculine would have and make based on the facts given:

- **You're forty-one and have been trying for four years.** If "it" was going to happen, it would have happened by now. At best you have a year—after that, *it's time to quit.*

- **You've done a bunch of treatments and tried a bunch of "kooky" things, but none of that witchcraft has worked.** The writing is on the wall. *If medicine can't help, nothing will.*

- **Your doctor says you have a less than 15% chance of getting pregnant.** What the doctor's really saying is you have an 85% chance of failing. Those are terrible odds; you might as well take your money to Las Vegas. Do you know what you could have done with $75k? If people found out how much money you've spent, they'd think you were crazy. You aren't spending any more. You want to retire someday!

- **You're drawn to my coaching but don't know if you should move forward with it.** What's some coach going to help you do that a doctor can't? *(Your masculine just happens to be ignorant of the fact that I'm*

*the fertility coach physicians turn to when THEY
struggle to conceive...)*

It's probably obvious where you'd end up with the masculine driving your decision bus. It's all about not looking stupid, cutting your losses, and caring a lot about what other people think. Any consideration for how you feel? Nope! It's about numbers, time, and what's "sensible." At no point is there any attention given to the fact that you are trying to have a f*cking baby, not negotiating the purchase of a car.

With the masculine in the driver's seat, you are very quickly headed to Fertility Quitsville, USA. You aren't likely to get a third, fourth, or fifth opinion, give yourself more time, explore creative solutions, take bigger risks, trust yourself (because the masculine reminds you of your failures as a defense mechanism), or, most importantly, *believe* having a baby is possible for you! As far as your masculine is concerned, it's just a matter of time before you throw in the towel and give up.

The Power of Feminine Contrast

To demonstrate the difference in the character and quality of decisions fueled by the feminine, we'll take that same set of facts given above and run it through what we'll call the Femme-O-Meter for fun. As a starting point, the feminine is possibility- and abundance-oriented. She sees beyond statistics and arbitrary limits. The feminine is a compassionate advocate rather than a finger-pointing blamer. She's all about another chance, bridging gaps, and the courage to believe. She uses her experience to discern instead of doubt. She's tapped into her intuition and knows it doesn't fail her when she leans in. She's gentle with mistakes and understands that they are guides in the right direction. So here's what I know she'd say:

- **You're forty-one and have been trying for four years.** Forty-one is the perfect time to have a baby. You've never been more prepared, mature, or financially stable. You finally have time to be a mom! *Keep going, baby; you know at least five other women who had babies in their forties!*

- **You've done a bunch of treatments and tried a bunch of "kooky" things, but none of that witchcraft has worked.** Look, babe, plenty of women who've had failed fertility treatments go on to have babies. Treatments aren't guarantees; they are opportunities. Let's find experts who believe in you to help figure this out. You always find a way.

- **Your doctor says you have a less than 15% chance of getting pregnant.** Fifteen percent means there's still a chance. You can always make more money. We are talking about your baby—who can put a price tag on that? Sure, $75k feels like a lot right now, but you'd invest ten times that to hear your baby call you "mama"! Who the hell retires these days, anyway?

- **You're drawn to fertility coaching but don't know if you should move forward with it.** You might have reached medicine's limit, but you haven't reached *your limit.* You know there's more to baby-making than just a sperm and egg coming together. Get that Fearlessly Fertile lady to help you clear your blocks and start fresh. You know you're meant to be a mom.

It's not much of a stretch to see that decisions from the feminine are going to keep you in the baby-making game. It's about what's true for you on the inside. The feminine is the part of you that knows you couldn't live with yourself if you gave up on the dream of being a mom, even if no one else around you gets it. The feminine urges you to believe and make decisions from what you desire, not what you fear. Influenced by the feminine, you aren't likely to give up. Here's what you'd do instead: shore up your mindset, allow yourself to receive the love and support you need, learn to believe in your body, and allow yourself to be in the peace and surrender that comes with expectation, not fear.

It's a Dance, Not Domination

When your thoughts and beliefs are aligned in positive possibility and you match them with bold, decisive action, the quality of your decisions improves dramatically, as does your results. This is the dance between the masculine and feminine that's required for success on this journey—you can see this play out in my story and in the stories of the women I've helped. The masculine supports the feminine, and the feminine informs the masculine. When you let the feminine in, your outlook improves, your energy goes up, you engage in self-care, you receive the support you need without judgment, and you look at yourself and your body in an entirely different way. You make nourishing your mind and body a priority, instead of just running yourself into the ground from exhaustion. *When you are different, your results are different.*

You needn't look any further than your own life to see the wreckage wrought by a dominant masculine. You are successful to a point, but you keep hitting a wall. To break through, you need the feminine. Your feminine will show you the whole truth, based on your intuition and what's in your heart, guided by faith and what feels right. Your feminine is the source of the trust you crave as you make your way to your baby. Wise women will take this information from the feminine to their masculine, and their masculine will execute. This is the interplay between the masculine and the feminine that I told you about earlier. When we allow the masculine to dominate without influence from the feminine, it's like trying to run a marathon with one leg. Sh*t gets hard real fast.

The Impact Isn't Just the Feels; It's Biological and Physical

When stuck in the masculine, you might be tempted to think, "I see what you're saying, Rosanne—the examples make sense to me when it comes to the 'feels'—but how is any of that really going to improve my chances of getting pregnant?" Simple. When you are stuck in your masculine, that creates stress. That stress creates a physiological response in your body, which, suppresses all nonessential body functions, including fertility. It's common knowledge that stress can cause disease and heart attacks. If stress can disrupt a basic life function, such as your heart beating to keep you alive, how could something as complex as fertility be immune? It's not. The data I will show you in chapter 7 proves it. But in order for you to fully understand the magnitude of the stress I'm talking about here that results from being disconnected with your feminine, you've got to see the full reach of that disconnect.

Let's review the math together. When you are disconnected from your feminine:

- Your boundaries are poor.
- You don't ask for what you truly want.
- You say yes when you mean no.
- You overwork.
- You under-receive.
- You are trapped in lack and scarcity.
- You focus on failure.
- You allow your contributions at work to be overlooked.
- You buy the lie that you have to suffer for success.
- You permit overwhelm to be a frequent visitor.

- You constantly compare yourself to coworkers, friends, family, and anyone you suspect may be more fertile than you.
- You live under the tyranny of an arbitrary, fear-based timeline.
- Your self-care is almost nonexistent.
- Your thoughts are consumed with doubt.
- You put yourself last.
- Your sex is soulless and mechanical.
- You can't remember the last time you felt pure, unadulterated joy.

With the education I have given you in the previous chapters, I am sure you could add another hundred ways your disconnection from your feminine is currently playing out in your life. You can't look at that list and seriously think to yourself that this soul-crushing stress stack is your run-of-the-mill occasional rough day. You've carried this for years. Your organs are sitting in this suck-ass soup. The weight of these stressors isn't merely an inconvenience; it's an invitation for illness. Just think about what this constant undercurrent of stress is doing to you. *And what's it doing to your fertility?*

If this masculine stress-mess math didn't get your attention, I will share more details about the data researchers have collected on the impact of stress on fertility and fertility outcomes in chapter 7.

Feminine Disconnect = Spiritual Disconnect

You don't have to be religious to understand that there is a spiritual component to conceiving. There is an X factor involved in the process that we may never fully understand. You can put sperm and an egg together and not get an embryo. You can transfer a poor quality embryo that yields a perfectly healthy baby. The creation of life isn't purely mechanical. It's more than random chance. It's miraculous.

When we are disconnected from our feminine, faith and miracles are hard to fathom. But any woman who wants to get to the end of her journey with a baby in her arms needs both. Over the ten-plus years that I have been doing this work, I've observed that grasping the spiritual aspect of fertility success is the hardest for women trapped in their masculine, and yet they are the ones that seem to crave it the most. I believe they know there's a spiritual aspect to conceiving, but the masculine will tell them that all this spiritual mumbo-jumbo is just superstition and what they really need to do is focus on the "facts." The problem is that material facts alone aren't enough on this journey. There is so much that we are just now beginning to understand, and we've barely scratched the surface. Faith and connection to the knowing in your heart that there is a baby for you bridges the gap between science and miracles. Without the feminine, it's difficult to have faith. The feminine is the conduit through which we connect with GUS. This connection is beyond the realm of the physical and isn't confined by the rules in the material world. For millennia, humans have described GUS as energy, love, and light. If you struggle with this, consider that scientists have been able to observe a "flash of light" at the moment of conception.[1] Scientists have explained this as being sparks of zinc released at the time a sperm meets an egg, [2] and while indeed that may be true, when connected to your feminine and your faith, you understand that the flash of light signals so much more than that—so let's go there.

I have noticed that women connected to their feminine can

---

1. Sarah Knapton, "Bright Flash of Light Marks Incredible Moment Life Begins When Sperm Meets Egg," Telegraph (UK), April 26, 2016, https://www.telegraph.co.uk/science/2016/04/26/bright-flash-of-light-marks-incredible-moment-life-begins-when-s/.

2. Knapton, "Bright Flash."

feel the presence of their babies. They see signs of their babies all around. When they visualize their lives with their babies, they quite literally feel the truth of their vision in their bodies, to the point that they shed tears. I've been present with women who tap into this part of themselves, and the energy is as palpable as it is powerful—it's moved me to tears as an observer, because we can feel truth when we are in the presence of it. Without the feminine connection to the spiritual, we lack access to a set of tools that help us connect with and bring the babies we know are meant for us into the physical world. *Come on!* Admit it—even the biggest skeptics have been drawn to stories of women who "just knew" and miraculously had babies, despite overwhelming odds.

As I described earlier, I knew with every fiber of my being that my son Asher was coming. I had no reason based in logic or on paper to believe it. It was something I felt in my heart. By opening up to my feminine and therefore opening up to the spiritual, I could tap into that knowing that only others open to their own spirituality can fully understand. I have watched similar transformations in the women I serve as well. Once they open up to their feminine and, in turn, explore their spiritual connection, feelings, signs, and a sense of knowing that never fails them begin showing up in their lives. If you listen to my podcast, you will hear every single one of the Miracle Mamas talk about how they "just knew," and when they trusted this spiritual aspect of themselves (which revealed itself in many forms), their babies followed shortly thereafter.

When you understand that disconnection from your feminine causes you to make fear-based choices that suck, creates toxic stress that is detrimental to your fertility, and denies you access to the realm of the spiritual, from which all miracles come, you can see why unf*cking your feminine is essential to your success.

It's Not Your Fault; The System Is Rigged

Now that you understand the hardcore upside of connecting to your feminine, there's a natural tendency, especially among success-oriented, high-achieving, hate-to-miss-sh*t women like us, to think, "How the hell did I miss this? How did I not see this? I'm a woman. Shouldn't this be obvious?"

Breathe, baby, breathe! There's something you need to know.

This destructive disconnection from the feminine is so pervasive and consistent among women of my generation and younger that there's no question in my mind that there's been a concerted effort to masculinize and distract women from their feminine nature. It isn't until a woman struggles with something as basic as her fertility that she becomes aware of the silent war that's been waged against her.

I am aware of how this sounds. The idea that generations of women could be manipulated out of their femininity to such a degree that they subordinate their desire for babies and families in favor of masculine measures of "success" sounds preposterous and, dare I say, conspiratorial. It's neither. *No, it's exactly what happened.* Women are living in the aftermath of this reality now. I was one of them. So are you.

I want to assure you that none of this is your fault. Even better? There are things you can do about it. I have practical solutions for you, but before we get into them, I believe that sharing some of the history of how we got to this point will empower you to recognize the masculine paradigm's influence in your own life, call it out when you see it, and not get trapped in it again moving forward. When you understand how women got so disconnected from the feminine, you will better understand the solutions I propose and why they are so radically effective.

If there's any part of you that still thinks the feminine can't be that important or that exploring your feminine is too much work, that's fine. You get to think what you want. But this information has helped women get and stay pregnant when no medical treatment could, at ages they were told made it "impossible." My ladies and I have our babies. *You don't.* If you want to change that so one day you can kiss your baby's toes, keep reading.

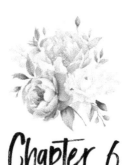

Chapter 6

WTF? How Did We Get So Far Away from Our Feminine?

The brief history I am sharing with you here has one purpose: to explain the steady progression of defeminizing women in American culture, which has wreaked havoc on women's self-image, wrecked our health and fertility, and at the same time systematically destroyed our families. I know that doesn't exactly sound like light reading, but stick with me here. When you understand how this happened, you can spot it playing out in your own life, and stop its evil rot from festering in your life and f*cking with your fertility.

The war on femininity started decades ago. Until you began feeling its effects, you would've had no clue it was going on. Consistent and cumulative attacks on your femininity have had the built-in anesthetic of being labeled "progress," so unless you had a super aware female relative in your family as your mentor, there's virtually no way you could have avoided being a casualty. You might have had a chance if you were raised in a home that taught and valued the roles of the traditional masculine and feminine, having no contact with the mainstream media, television, public schools, government officials, organized religion, standard American healthcare, or just about every other juggernaut influence in modern life. But even then, once you set foot outside that bubble, *BOOM!* And absent those circumstances, you would've had no idea that the propaganda you were being fed from every direction, cloaked in claims of "progress" and liberation, was poison.

If you were born after 1970 and didn't grow up under the proverbial rock I just described, you can be almost 100% sure defeminization has its greasy fingerprints all over your life, and you are definitely not alone.

Presupposition of "Progress"

"Progress" for our purposes here means a masculinized ideal for women that is a near-complete repudiation of traditionally feminine roles, attitudes, and sensibilities. The idea behind this is that women in traditionally feminine roles, with traditionally feminine attitudes and sensibilities, are oppressed and have a poor quality of life. The solution, which is posed as "progress," would be for women to escape their oppression by becoming more like men. The only way for a woman to do so is by pursuing higher education, working outside the home, and having an income stream separate from that of her husband or partner. If a woman isn't doing those specific things, she's not living to her highest potential, is trapped in a mediocre life, and *quick, somebody help her!* The idea is that for women to be making "progress" and be "liberated," they must be freed from the bondage of domesticity. This notion of "progress" is one-sided, though. Rather than being built on a premise of legitimate choice, it presumes that pursuits other than higher education, career, and financial independence are inferior. Within this presumption is the idea that *if* a woman decides to step into a feminine role as a mother or homemaker, it will only happen after she has an education and career, and the deviation from her path of masculine achievement will only be temporary.

We will certainly get into more about this later, but for now, I want you have a clear point of reference when I refer to "progress."

After nearly three generations of American women being force-fed the idea that their femininity was a liability and a virtual guarantee of subjugation, we have reached a warped "new normal" for women in this country. American women are currently struggling more with fertility than ever before. We've never been more unhappy, our intimate relationships are a mess, and we wonder why we are so medicated, unfulfilled, overwhelmed, burned out, and disillusioned.

Some women wake up to this reality through the gift of a major health or personal crisis. Many get glimpses of it through some nagging but amorphous feeling of malaise but go back to sleep, thinking, "Nah, that couldn't be me. I'm doing *okay*," which is really code for "I'm numb." Sadly, most never wake up at all. Sadly, we were sold a fairy tale of progress that, in the end, has benefited few and betrayed the women it claimed to promote and protect.

The Propaganda of Perennial Patriarchal Progress

While there is evidence that the attack on femininity in the United States started much earlier than the events I will describe here, there was a series of events starting in the early 1960s that presents an undeniable line of demarcation from which it moved from covert to brazenly overt. With President John F. Kennedy in the White House, Jacqueline Kennedy as First Lady, and the Camelot mythology in full swing, this was the last time the American public was served up an image at a national level of a decidedly feminine figure as an ideal. Young, beautiful, well-educated, self-possessed, multilingual, an accomplished journalist in her own right, fashionable, a doting mother, and still traditionally feminine, Jackie Kennedy was an icon as what I call a *Beacon of Both*. She was both personally empowered and feminine. Certainly, one could call into question how empowered she was for myriad reasons and depending on which rumors or innuendo you believe, but, by the same token, it was patently obvious that she was no ditsy damsel in distress. Despite the breathy hush of her voice, there was a steely-eyed strength in her countenance that let everyone know she wasn't a pushover.

At this time in American history, being Jackie-esque was the feminine ideal. Even a cursory online search of media, advertising, and demographic data from the 1950s and early 1960s shows women decidedly feminine in appearance and in the focus of their pursuits and purpose. While it's true that the demand for labor during World War II had ushered in a dramatic increase in the number of women in the workforce—adding 6.5 million women to the existing 13 million who were already working outside the home by 1940[1]—once the war was over, women went back to their roles as wives and mothers in droves. Between 1950 and 1960, close to 70% of women were married, just over 10% were widowed, less than 5% were divorced, and the number of women who had never been married fell to less than 20%.[2] By the time Kennedy took office

---

1. Pavithra Mohan, "This Pandemic Isn't the First Time Women Have Left the Workforce in Droves," *Fast Company*, March 29, 2021, https://www.fastcompany.com/90617765/this-pandemic-isnt-the-first-time-women-have-left-the-work force-in-droves.

2. "Figure MS-1b: Women's Marital Status," in *Decennial Censuses, 1950 to 1990, and Current Population Survey, Annual Social and Economic Supplements, 1993 to 2023*, U.S. Census Bureau, last updated November 21, 2023, https://www.census.gov/content/dam/Census/library/visualizations/time-series/demo/families-and-households/ms-1b.pdf.

in 1961, the United States was well into the baby boom, a record number of births between 1946 and 1964.[3] Between those years, the US saw nearly 76 million babies born, which was an increase of more than 50% over the population in 1945.[4] By 1960, the average number of babies born per woman was 3.443,[5] and 4,257,850 babies were born that year alone.[6] What's even more interesting is that this focus on the family and the home held firm despite women attending college in higher numbers[7] and participating in the workforce outside of the home at a rate of nearly 40% by 1960.[8]

While not every woman of that era aspired to "be like Jackie," or at least like the image of her that was widely portrayed, these numbers demonstrate that by 1960, women were making advancements in their education and outside-the-home employment without necessarily having to abandon the desires, pursuits, and affinities that made them feminine. Femininity was natural, good, inoffensive, and, compared to where I believe women stand today, *a wonderfully liberating given.* Working was something more women were choosing to do, which in and of itself was neither masculine nor feminine—it was simply a choice. But what makes the nature of the choice to work in the '60s different from that same choice today is that it

---

3. Philip Bump, "Baby Boomer," *Encyclopedia Britannica*, last updated November 12, 2023, https://www.britannica.com/topic/baby-boomers.

4. Bump, "Baby Boomer."

5. "U.S. Fertility Rate 1950–2023," MacroTrends, accessed November 26, 2023, https://www.macrotrends.net/countries/USA/united-states/fertility-rate.

6. B. E. Hamilton et al., "Natality Trends in the United States, 1909–2018," National Center for Health Statistics, last updated July 12, 2018, https://www.cdc.gov/nchs/data-visualization/natality-trends/index.htm.

7. Claudia Golden, Lawrence F. Katz, and Ilyana Kuziemko, "The Homecoming of American College Women: The Reversal of the College Gender Gap," *Journal of Economic Perspectives* 20, no. 4 (2006): 133–56, https://doi.org/10.1257/jep.24.3.i.

8. "Changes in Men's and Women's Labor Force Participation Rates," U.S. Bureau of Labor Statistics, January 10, 2007, https://www.bls.gov/opub/ted/2007/jan/wk2/art03.htm.

didn't come at the price of one's femininity. The early 1960s, prior to the "women's movement," were a time when women could be in the workplace without necessarily having to look like a man or take on masculine traits. We see this demonstrably in women's workwear from that time, which was still traditionally feminine.[9]

To be clear, I am not in any way holding up this period of American history as some kind of social, cultural, legal, or moral ideal. There were unquestionably horrific injustices of all hair-raising varieties perpetrated against women of that time. Sexual abuse, domestic violence, and gender discrimination went largely unreported, unprosecuted, and without just resolution. Married women couldn't even have bank accounts without their husbands' signatures or get loans on their own until the Equal Credit Opportunity Act was passed by Congress in 1974.[10] It would be decades before women would see the long-overdue advances in civil rights that we deserved, and arguably, the advancement of our civil rights is a process that continues today. But the early 1960s represent a critical turning point, as they were the last time when a woman could freely and openly express the feminine in all aspects of her life without a carefully coordinated multifront culture war screaming in her face that she was weak, uninformed, and, more importantly, *wrong* for doing so. A wolf-in-sheep's-clothing pivot was about to take place under the guise of "progress," one that the granddaughters and great-granddaughters of these women would pay dearly for decades later.

---

9. Amy Woods, "Fashion Empowers Ambition: The Evolution of Women's Workwear," The Women's Network, accessed April 11, 2024, https://www.thewomens.network/blog/fashion-empowers-ambition-the-evolution-of-womens-workwear.

10. Jamela Adam, "When Could Women Open a Bank Account?," Forbes Advisor, last updated May 20, 2023, https://www.forbes.com/advisor/banking/when-could-women-open-a-bank-account/.

The Scam of Success Being a Masculine Game

A guiding principle of the attack on femininity is the notion that the feminine is insufficient and weak. Since the 1960s, around the time of the so-called "women's movement," the mainstream message we got about what it meant to be "feminist" was essentially and ironically anti-feminine.

Before I go any further, I want to make a clear distinction about how I will use the terms *feminist/feminism* moving forward. I see feminism as the belief that women and men have equal rights under constitutional, common, and natural law. Therefore, a feminist, under the definition I have given, is someone who believes and agrees with that statement—no activism required; it's simply a belief. When you see me use the term "feminist" or "feminism" in quotation marks, I am pointing to the black hole of a zillion and five mutations of my basic working definition of feminism. When I use "feminist" or "feminism" in quotes, I am pointing to definitions that have metastasized into meanings that incorporate divisive political bias and have hijacked the conversation about women having equal rights under the law—not *more* rights, *equal* rights. That insane discussion could be a book of its own, and I will not delve into it here. I believe the feminine is powerful enough on her own that she doesn't need politics—*she deserves awareness and understanding.*

So, back to our discussion of how "feminism" became anti-feminine.

Since the time of "women's lib," a concerted effort has been made by media and interest groups to masculinize women. We were encouraged to think and act more like men, particularly when it comes to success in the workplace. The idea was that to "compete" with men, we had to be like men. Women were bombarded by their alleged movement's messaging that the natural inclinations and characteristics we have as women weren't enough. Women were told success required them to be "more." That *more*, as you will see, translated into *masculine*. The promise behind these ideas, largely espoused by second-wave "feminists" such as Betty Friedan, was that by escaping the cage of domesticity through educational and career advancement, women would be happier, achieve greater personal fulfillment, and have drastically improved quality of life.[11] But, as you will see in chapter 7, this was a promise with a devastatingly poor payoff.

One of the most visible demonstrations of *masculine is more* was the rejection of being classically feminine in appearance. Google the change in fashion during this period, and you'll notice the masculinization of women's clothing, particularly in the workplace. It wasn't until the late '60s and early '70s that we saw women wearing pants and masculine pantsuits at work (other than rare times when safety required it).[12] This shift in fashion coincides with a changing narrative about women in the workforce and what it takes to be "successful," which we will unpack in a moment.[13] This change continued into the late '70s and '80s with women's "power suits."[14] An entire generation of women were damned to go to work looking like NFL linebackers!

This masculinization extended beyond the battle cry of "anything a man can do, a woman can do!" and dressing more masculinely; it also twisted into a weird message that women should prove they could do it all at home and at work, with no help, every day, tirelessly, and yet still exude a feminine allure. It was another way of saying, "You want to show how powerful you are? Do it all! And do it yourself!" I distinctly remember a

11. "Betty Friedan," *Encyclopedia Britannica*, last updated March 5, 2024, https://www.britannica.com/biography/Betty-Friedan.
12. Woods, "Fashion Empowers Ambition."
13. Woods, "Fashion Empowers Ambition."
14. Woods, "Fashion Empowers Ambition."

series of commercials that came out in the late '70s and continued into the '80s for a perfume called Enjoli. In the commercials, the female protagonist proclaimed things like, " 'Cause I'm a woman! I can bring home the bacon! Fry it up in a pan. And never let you forget you're a man!"[15] Thus, the "feminist" Frankenstein's monster of the superwoman was born—the antithetical nightmare of the traditional feminine ruthlessly released on the American public. The imagery was an invitation for women to trade their femininity for a distinctly masculine energy that morphed them into "liberated," man-eating, workaholic porn stars who wore cheap perfume and delighted in full-time work, household chores, taking care of the kids, and being insatiable sex kittens, all at the same time. *Can you smell the progress?* Women may have gained more access to educational and professional opportunities, but they'd have to pursue them while still maintaining the other full-time jobs they had at home with their families. *It's the sweet sound of liberation! Can you hear it?*

American advertisers loved this superwoman ideal, which set women up for a new level of consumerism that led them to believe they could "have it all" *if they did it all*—and bought all the books, magazines, and clothes that would get them there.[16] This was yet another blow to the feminine, as it kept women in a masculine state of chasing and proving. Women were propagandized to chase and prove they could live up to an ideal that was highly stylized and unquestionably cooked up by a man, an ideal that trapped them in a no-win game.[17] Seriously, only

15. "Enjoli Perfume – 'Cause I'm A Woman....' (Commercial, 1982)," The Museum of Classic Chicago Television, January 5, 2018, YouTube video, 0:31, https://youtu.be/3N9K7eoVtmo?si=IPaelDHJkuoi_EEl. This version of the ad originally aired on local Chicago TV on Wednesday, December 1, 1982.
16. Ruth Rosen, "Who Said 'We Could Have It All'?," openDemocracy, August 2, 2012, https://www.opendemocracy.net/en/5050/who-said-we-could-have-it-all/.
17. Rosen, "Have It All."

a dude would be nuts enough to try to sell the idea that you could work all day, take care of the kids, cook a delectable meal, and then be a voracious vixen in the sack!

The Masculine Mommy Wars

The notion of the superwoman persists today and can be seen in a different form through the so-called "Mommy Wars." This psychological sabotage basically pits working moms and stay-at-home moms against each other in a battle over who is the better mom or who's "the mommiest."[18] I've witnessed this insanity firsthand, and it is gross. I see this as another manifestation of the masculinization of women; it incites the need for women to compete and prove their "enoughness." It just moves the fighting from the workplace to the school pickup line! So much for celebrating a sister's choice. We have working moms looking down on stay-at-home moms as squanderers of their talents, while the "Stay at Homes" scoff at working moms who haven't crafted 100% organic cupcakes for Billy's birthday, topped with buttercream frosting they churned themselves from the Jersey cows they milked that morning! Where's the loving, supportive community that some "feminist" messaging promised?

Thanks to the Mommy Wars, we can see this weird offshoot of "feminism" that vilifies the idea that you can have it all—meaningful work and a family. The idea is that you can only be good at one, so you must *pick*. It's total and complete nonsense; reject it. As an individual, you get to create your own mix based on your own values. It's the feminine way. Anyone who tells you that you must choose is just mad at the choice they made, and they want you to be just as miserable as they are.

---

18. Rosen, "Have It All."

Masculinization into the New Millennium

The masculinization of women continued to be part of the mainstream narrative well into the 2000s and morphed into girlboss "feminism"—aka "liberal feminism"—in the 2010s.[19] What's interesting about this next phase in the attack on femininity is it didn't just push the idea of women advancing by being in the workplace; since, by the 2000s, having a job was a given, it upped the ante by being unabashedly elitist in its cliquishness. It was a worship of rich, powerful female politicians and CEOs—completely ignoring women who chose to be mothers, weren't rich, and didn't care for pantsuits.[20] Girlboss "feminism" was all about hardcore hustle and a spider-monkey-like ascent of the corporate ladder, with little concern for uplifting women as a group.[21] There was an underlying aggression to this ethos that was a continuation and amplification of the man-eater "Enjoli" image I mentioned before—except now this superwoman was affluent. The widely detested poster girl for girlboss psychopathic "feminism" was Elizabeth Holmes,[22] former CEO of the defunct Theranos,[23] who bilked investors out of more than $450 million dollars.[24] The girlboss image wasn't connected to everyday women; the quintessential girl-

---

19. Liza Featherstone, "Is It Just Us, or Is Girl-Boss Feminism Waning?," *Jacobin*, September 26, 2023, https://jacobin.com/2023/09/liberal-feminism-girl-boss-decline-hillary-clinton-one-percent.
20. "Is It Just Us?"
21. Zoe Luu, "The Irony of #Girlboss Feminism," The Women's Network, May 26, 2022, https://www.thewomens.network/blog/the-irony-of-girlboss-feminism.
22. Eden Bouvier, "Elizabeth Holmes and The Case of Feminism," Write Like a Girl, Medium, March 21, 2022, https://medium.com/write-like-a-girl/elizabeth-holmes-and-the-case-of-feminism-a-particularly-interesting-case-study-e4ff54d4b489.
23. Martha Gill, " 'Girlboss' Used to Suggest a Kind of Role Model. How Did it Become a Sexist Putdown?," *Guardian* (US), August 21, 2022, https://www.theguardian.com/commentisfree/2022/aug/21/girlboss-used-to-suggest-role-model-sexist-putdown.
24. Kari Paul, "Elizabeth Holmes Objects to $250 Monthly Payments to Ther-

boss upped the masculinity factor and had an attitude toward femininity and motherhood that sounded a hell of a lot like *"You poor thing."*[25] This warped progeny of the women's movement is yet another example of how women are consistently being sold the idea that standing in their feminine isn't enough —and no woman will be enough until she's pretty much a man!

Wait! Wasn't feminism supposed to be about equal rights and getting out from underneath the patriarchy? Isn't this nonsense just asking us to become part of it?

When was the last time you saw the feminine celebrated in your workplace, where women were encouraged to nurture each other's success and women's natural emotions and rhythms weren't demonized? I never saw that sh*t when I was a deputy district attorney, and *I worked in an office where there were loads of women in top positions.* In fact, we all knew that if you wanted to be taken seriously, you had better not show any emotion, and if you dared to go out on maternity leave, chances were you weren't going back to the plum assignment you had worked your ass off for. Was that the written or stated policy? Of course not. That wouldn't be legal. But in my opinion, the undercurrent was crystal clear. The idea that women must behave in masculine or aggressive ways to succeed didn't stop when it came to the workplace or overachieving at home. It also showed up in the landscape of both sexual and familial relationships between men and women.

As the Feminine Fell, the Nuclear Family Destabilized

As traditional feminine roles took a backseat to a more masculine ideal and the birthrate in the United States by the late

---

anos Victims," *Guardian* (US), June 14, 2023, https://www.theguardian.com/us-news/2023/jun/14/elizabeth-holmes-theranos-victims-repayment-objection.
25. Featherstone, "Girl-Boss Feminism."

1970s had plummeted to half of what it had been in 1960,[26] the nuclear family in the United States was about to take hits from three new directions. The first struck at the institution of marriage itself on September 5, 1969, when California governor Ronald Reagan signed no-fault divorce legislation into law, the first law of its kind in this country.[27] Prior to this legislation, a husband or wife had to make an allegation of "fault" by their spouse in order to be granted a dissolution of the marriage. This meant that the spouse asking for the divorce had to prove their spouse "did" something—adultery, abandonment, cruelty, felony conviction, or other unsavory behaviors.[28] No-fault divorce opened the floodgates to couples filing for divorce; now they could split up on the basis of "irreconcilable differences" rather than enduring the expense, theatrics, and misery of a long, drawn-out proceeding, hoping with bated breath that a judge would be convinced enough to grant their divorce.[29] Divorce rates immediately skyrocketed in the 1970s, with 71.4% of filings being made by women; rates later declined throughout the rest of the 1980s.[30]

At first blush, this sounds like emancipation and freedom, but the facts I will share both in the rest of this chapter and in the next raise serious questions about whether changing the landscape of families and catapulting women into taking on the role of head of household were all they were cracked up to be.

26. "U.S. Fertility Rate 1950–2023."

27. Donna S. Hershkowitz and Drew R. Liebert, *The Direction of Divorce Reform in California: From Fault to No-Fault...and Back Again?* (Sacramento, CA: Assembly Judiciary Committee, California State Legislature, 1997), https://ajud.assembly. ca.gov/sites/ajud.assembly.ca.gov/files/reports/1197%20divorcereform97.pdf.

28. Christy Bieber, "What Is a No Fault Divorce?," *Forbes*, July 26, 2023, https:// www.forbes.com/advisor/legal/divorce/no-fault-divorce/.

29. "Advance Report of Final Divorce Statistics, 1988," *Monthly Vital Statistics Report* 39, no. 12 (May 21, 1991), https://doi.org/10.18356/3023d8cd-en.

30. "Advance Report of Final Divorce Statistics, 1988."

Women Left Home for the Office, Changing the Landscape of Both

From an economic standpoint, the nuclear family also took a hit with rising inflation that steadily took place starting in the early 1970s.[31] In 1960, 62% of American homes had a father who was the breadwinner, a stay-at-home mom, and one or more children,[32] but by the end of the 1970s, for the first time ever, more than half of women had jobs outside of the home. This was no longer simply a matter of women's liberation; it was also about making ends meet.[33] This without question had a direct impact on the family structure and the children in those families, as Mom was no longer home to care for them.[34] We see this most clearly in the rise of the latchkey kid, a phenomenon that arose in the 1970s and 1980s when the children known as Generation X "went through [their] all-important formative years as one of the least parented, least nurtured generations in U.S. history."[35] This not surprisingly coincides with the increasing divorce rates.[36]

Between families fractured by divorce and the US economy

---

31. Mitra Toossi and Teresa L. Morisi, "Women in the Workforce Before, During, and After the Great Recession: Spotlight on Statistics," U.S. Bureau of Labor Statistics, July 2017, https://www.bls.gov/spotlight/2017/women-in-the-workforce-before-during-and-after-the-great-recession/home.htm.

32. "Women in the Workforce: 1970s - A Decade of Change," HR & PEO Services for Small Business, October 20, 2022, https://www.propelhr.com/blog/women-in-the-workforce-1970s-a-decade-of-change-for-women.

33. "Women in the Workforce."

34. D'Vera Cohn, Gretchen Livingston, and Wendy Wang, "After Decades of Decline, A Rise in Stay-at Home Mothers," Pew Research Center, April 8, 2014, https://www.pewresearch.org/social-trends/2014/04/08/after-decades-of-decline-a-rise-in-stay-at-home-mothers/.

35. Susan Gregory Thomas, "All Apologies: Thank You for the 'Sorry,'" HuffPost, August 23, 2011, https://www.huffpost.com/entry/all-apologies-thank-you-f_b_931718.

36. Amy McKenna, "Generation X," *Encyclopedia Britannica*, March 1, 2024, https://www.britannica.com/topic/Generation-X.

in shambles, the American family in many different strata got rocked. While indeed women's independence and earning potential increased during this time, there have been grave and enduring consequences on family structure, femininity, and, ultimately, fertility that are impacting women today, which I will discuss further as we move forward.

While women and their families were adjusting to these changing conditions, the landscape of the workplace itself had to change to accommodate its increasingly female constituency. Post–World War II, most women didn't anticipate spending much of their time working outside of the home, but by the 1970s, that completely changed.[37] It was almost a given that women would spend significant time in the labor force, which led to an increase in women seeking training and education that would support careers instead of just getting random, go-nowhere jobs.[38] By 1978, legal measures were put in place to protect women from discrimination during pregnancy with the passage of the aptly named Pregnancy Discrimination Act.[39] There was also growing awareness around sexual harassment,[40] but it wasn't until much later that the issue was given the attention it deserves.

Since entering the workforce, women have struggled to earn the same wages as men for many different reasons that have been argued from many different positions, but the gap in earnings between genders has been narrowing over the decades as women have left typically female positions as clerical support, teachers, and nurses to pursue careers as doctors,

37. Janet L. Yellen, "The History of Women's Work and Wages and How it Has Created Success for Us All," Brookings, May 2020, https://www.brookings.edu/articles/the-history-of-womens-work-and-wages-and-how-it-has-created-success-for-us-all/.

38. Yellen, "Women's Work and Wages."

39. Yellen, "Women's Work and Wages."

40. Yellen, "Women's Work and Wages."

lawyers, professors, and other higher paying professions.[41] With these professions being historically overwhelmingly comprised of men, this was another circumstance under which women, in order to be accepted or to compete, had to present in a more masculine way. Most women who have been through law school, med school, or other professional schools, even recently, will agree that the energy in those environments is thoroughly masculine and that there isn't much room for the exercise of one's femininity. *I am one of those women!* The masculinization doesn't end in the professional schools, either; it's only further solidified once women get into their offices. Despite significant workplace advances and gains women have made in pay and opportunity, the overall expectation is that women will show up in their masculine.

Not So Feminine in Pop Culture

By the late 1960s, media and pop culture began perpetuating a very different image of femininity. As a child in the 1970s, I could see the stark contrast between *Leave It to Beaver*'s perfectly coiffed, never flustered June Cleaver and the female lead characters in shows like *The Mary Tyler Moore Show*, *Alice*, and *The Brady Bunch*. These new shows began portraying images the American public hadn't seen to the same degree on TV before: a single, career woman as a lead character,[42] a blue-collar single mom struggling to support her son,[43] and a

---

41. Yellen, "Women's Work and Wages."

42. "The Mary Tyler Moore Show," *Encyclopedia Britannica*, last updated January 25, 2024, https://www.britannica.com/topic/The-Mary-Tyler-Moore-Show.

43. Hilton Dresden, "Hollywood Flashback: 'Alice' Served Up a Hit for CBS in 1976," *Hollywood Reporter*, December 16, 2022, https://www.hollywoodreporter.com/tv/tv-news/hollywood-flashback-alice-cbs-1235283325/.

woman trying to navigate a blended family of six kids.[44] While they're relatively benign by today's over-the-top, rub-social-issues-in-your-face standards, these shows began normalizing themes of women in more masculine, breadwinner roles. Specifically, in the case of *The Brady Bunch*, we see Marcia Brady exploring her developing "feminism" by trying to join her brothers' Boy Scout troop and enduring feats of "manliness."[45] (Wait! Did you catch that? Another example of women needing to live up to a masculine paradigm—*to be equal, we should act like men!*) While the introduction of more "feminist" themes was done with a lighter touch, during the same time frame, we see traditionally feminine characters being increasingly parodied. This was most clearly seen with the perpetuation of the "dumb blond" stereotype up through the 1980s, where the decidedly feminine characters, almost exclusively blond, were made victims of their femininity and were usually bailed out by their more masculine, liberated brunette counterparts. To see this in action, consider an afternoon of a retro-TV watch party featuring shows like *Charlie's Angels*, *Three's Company*, and *Dallas*.

Men: The Real Winners of the Sexual Revolution

To fully understand the depth and range of the slow creep of masculinization of women in the United States, *we've got to talk about sex.* Specifically, the sexual revolution. Around the same time that women were gaining ground in the fight for equal rights in the 1960s, there was a parallel and related movement that is commonly referred to as the sexual revolution. The

---

44. "The Brady Bunch," *Encyclopedia Britannica*, November 17, 2023, https://www.britannica.com/topic/The-Brady-Bunch.
45. Jon Keller, "Keller @ Large: The Brady Bunch Changed How Americans Viewed Women," CBS News, July 12, 2011, https://www.cbsnews.com/boston/news/keller-large-the-brady-bunch-changed-how-americans-viewed-women/.

premise of this movement was to free people up to express themselves sexually outside the commonly accepted confines of marriage. The sexual revolution got a massive boost from the oral contraceptive pill being approved for use in the United States by the FDA on May 9, 1960,[46] and then later from the legalization of abortion with the United States Supreme Court ruling in *Roe v. Wade* in 1973.[47]

It's important to note that while there was some crossover between the women's movement and the sexual revolution, these were distinct social movements that didn't exactly stand for the same thing. In the simplest terms, one was about the rights of women, and the other was about loosening the social stigma about sex in general. Some saw the sexual revolution as furthering the empowerment of women,[48] but decades later, we can see that isn't the case.

As much as "feminists" would like you to believe that the sexual revolution was a big capital *w* Win for women, it's hands down the best thing to have happened to men. Think about it. With oral contraception readily available, abortion legal and celebrated, and relationships becoming more fleeting and transactional, who benefits? Men!

No longer saddled with the societal pressure or obligation to raise a child, since the women's movement has beaten the drum of "you don't need a man" for decades, women have been relegated to "undercutting" each other and competing for men —which leaves us sad, alone, and miserable.[49] The result is

---

46. Sarah McCammon, "How the Approval of the Birth Control Pill 60 Years Ago Helped Change Lives," Houston Public Media, May 9, 2020, https://www.houstonpublicmedia.org/npr/2020/05/09/852807455/how-the-approval-of-the-birth-control-pill-60-years-ago-helped-change-lives/.

47. "Roe v. Wade Is Decided, January 22, 1973," History.com, accessed April 11, 2024, https://www.history.com/this-day-in-history/roe-v-wade.

48. "The Pill and the Sexual Revolution," PBS, accessed April 11, 2024, https://www.pbs.org/wgbh/americanexperience/features/pill-and-sexual-revolution/.

49. Glenn T. Stanton, "The Pill: Did It Cause the Sexual Revolution?," Focus on

men having more access to sex for lower and lower levels of
commitment, thus making women weaker players in the field
and, arguably, therefore worse off.[50] *Winner, winner, chicken
dinner, men!*

Perhaps the craziest con of the alleged sexual revolution,
particularly for women, is that we were convinced to have sex
on masculine terms. Said another way, we were conned into
believing it's powerful and forward-thinking to have sex like
men. *There it is again!* Did you spot it? To have "progress," we
must be more like men. Sound familiar? Now, when I say *have
sex like men*, I believe the most accurate way to define that is in
terms of the casual, emotionless, transactional, no-strings-
attached attitude toward sex that is often attributed to men.[51]
It's an ethos of seeming nonattachment that is somehow
supposed to be more powerful or empowered.

Now, I don't care what kind of garbage you've been fed
about women being able to have sex like men; it simply isn't
true, and it completely denies biological and psychological
realities.[52] How many well-adjusted, high-functioning,
emotionally stable women with high self-esteem do you know
who try this? We've all known one woman in our social circle
who might be "that," but behind her bravado is a broken heart,
concealing the wounds she sustained from buying this lie. In
the late 1990s and early 2000s, at least the writers for Darren
Star's *Sex and the City* were honest about this with the character

the Family, July 6, 2010, https://www.focusonthefamily.com/marriage/the-pill-
did-it-cause-the-sexual-revolution/.

50. Stanton, "The Pill."

51. Tom Rasmussen, "I Couldn't Help But Wonder...Should Women Have Sex
Like Men?," *Vogue*, November 3, 2022, https://www.vogue.com/article/women-
sex-like-men.

52. Ruth C. White, "No Strings Attached Sex (NSA): Can Women Really Do
It?," *Psychology Today*, November 20, 2011, https://www.psychologytoday.com/
us/blog/culture-in-mind/201111/no-strings-attached-sex-nsa-can-women-really-
do-it.

Samantha Jones. Her Olympic sex drive and "sex like a man" antics were hilarious, but we could all see her pain and how she was her happiest when in a committed relationship. Just rewatch the series for characters Richard and Smith, and you'll see what I mean.

This weird and contorted, masculine approach to sex persists today with hookup-focused dating apps like Bumble and Hinge, "swipe culture," and women becoming significant consumers of pornography.[53] Sixty years on from the bellowing calls for women to be unshackled from sexual objectification, we find ourselves in a time when access to such material has never been more ubiquitous (it's anywhere you and your phone are) and arguably condoned by some "feminists" as freedom and progress, when in reality it's more like, *if you can't beat 'em, join 'em!* Is this really what "winning" as a woman looks like?

The presupposition here is that women *want* to have sex like men and that to be "equal" in the bedroom, a woman must get there on *man terms*. This is particularly preposterous in its application to a topic as intimate as sex. What this shows is that, even in how we approach our physical intimacy as women, we've been conditioned to find "progress" and power in the rejection of our feminine nature and biological predisposition to sex with emotion and attachment.[54] *Even our bedrooms provide no refuge from the masculine paradigm!*

Without the Feminine, Our Relationships Are F*cked Up

So, in this post-masculinization world, what happens when you

---

53. Michael Castleman, "This Is Why Many Women Watch Porn," Psychology Today, June 1, 2020, https://www.psychologytoday.com/us/blog/all-about-sex/202006/is-why-many-women-watch-porn.
54. Joe Malone, "What's Happening in Male vs. Female Brains During Sex?," Natural Womanhood, February 17, 2023, https://naturalwomanhood.org/what-happens-in-mens-vs-women-brains-during-sex/.

get past a hookup? It gets even more confusing—and this has left women wondering where all the *real men* went.

Yes, I said *real men*. Not the wishy-washy, afraid-of-their-own-shadow man-children that decades of emasculating American public education and media have churned out. The mainlined messaging we got from 1960s "feminism" is that men are dangerous oppressors by nature, so we need to reject traditional masculine traits of protection, provision, leadership, and strength to embrace a softer, gentler man who is more "sensitive and caring"—one who we can dominate. Here we are again! It's the same annoyingly boring play of switching roles with men, *then becoming one.* I bet you're starting to catch on to the con.

This messaging lacks consideration of what women desire —what happened to being equals? Does equal necessarily mean "same"? For a woman to be an equal in her relationship, is she required to emasculate her man? Can't men and women lead from their unique strengths without having to abandon what makes them who they are? It makes sense to me that, as power gets redistributed or restructured in a relationship, there may be initial pendulum swings in either direction, but judging from what I see in my coaching practice, have experienced in my own life, and observe in society, the pendulum hasn't found its center.

What I see today are generations of women brought up under programming that's told them the feminine is weak, who buy into a masculinized ideal, become wildly successful in the workplace, are earning six and seven figures in their professions and businesses, and have brass balls outside the home but struggle to connect in their relationships as equals in their *feminine.* We know one mode, and that's *Man Mode.* Then we wonder why our needs aren't being met in our intimate relationships. I see amazing powerhouse women end up with men they often outpace in education, earning, or both.[55] Then they get frustrated with those men for not being better providers or for not being "man enough." I witness this playing out almost every day in my coaching practice. Women who achieve success under the masculine paradigm in this country do not want that same paradigm operating in their homes.[56] The problem is that we are so disconnected from our feminine that we don't know how to be feminine in our relationships. We attract men into our lives who are masculine, and we find ourselves meeting their masculine with our own masculine, which is an absolute disaster. Why? Because when we are stuck in our masculine, we don't tell our men what we really need, we struggle to express how we *really* feel, we over-give, we are constantly doing, and then we get angry because we are exhausted and our needs aren't being met. See the problem? We are in Man Mode with our men!

I tell my ladies all the time, "If you approach your man from masculine energy, he will treat you like a man!" How can he care for, protect, and nurture you when he can't see that you need those things? I know that decades of masculine programming may have you take issue with the "protect" part of what I just said, but I'm sorry—deep down, you know you want to know that your man will protect and advocate for you. There is no shame in that, and you are certainly not alone.[57] Wanting those things doesn't make you weak. Nor does it mean you can

55. Ludmila Leiva, "Rejected for Being 'Too Successful,' Career-Driven Women Say It's Better to Know," Refinery29, September 25, 2018, https://www.refinery29.com/en-us/successful-women-dating-men.
56. Suzanne Venker, "Why Super-Successful Women Struggle in Love," *Washington Examiner*, October 9, 2019, https://www.washingtonexaminer.com/opinion/1823575/why-super-successful-women-struggle-in-love/.
57. Paul Joannides, "What Women Want in a Man," Psychology Today, November 1, 2023, https://www.psychologytoday.com/us/blog/as-you-like-it/202310/what-women-want-in-a-man/.

no longer be a card-carrying feminist.[58] It's part of your feminine nature to desire love and protection! Embrace that. That desire isn't some throwback to the 1950s, either; it's biological, and it's also why we even tend to prefer more masculine-looking men.[59] Many women think they have to settle for beta-male Ross from *Friends* when, in truth, they crave Rip from *Yellowstone*. Trusting your feminine in your intimate relationship will allow you to be smarter and ultimately more fulfilled than that.

Mass Masculinization Confused Our Roles and Muted Our Voices

Not only has anti-feminine cultural programming confused women about what we really want in men, but it has made a mess of the roles we have in our homes and strangely silenced our voices. The superwoman ideal we discussed earlier is still pervasive today, albeit with a more subdued style and appearance, and now she's paired with a more compliant generation of men beaten down by "feminist" rhetoric. While there's no doubt from a practical standpoint that women can do it all, *nobody's asking if they should!* This has led to women taking on massive responsibilities in the workplace, at home, and in their relationships while asking for little to no help and, when they do, feeling shame for it. Because that would be—dare I say it? —*weak!* The result of this craziness is that we have millions of American women running around exhausted, overwhelmed, and, despite their professional accomplishments, feeling

58. Shannon Lell, "I'm a Feminist Who's Attracted to 'Manly Men,' " *Washington Post*, September 13, 2016, https://www.washingtonpost.com/news/soloish/wp/2016/09/13/im-a-feminist-whos-attracted-to-manly-men/.

59. Urszula M. Marcinkowska et al., "Women's Preferences for Men's Facial Masculinity Are Strongest Under Favorable Ecological Conditions," *Scientific Reports* 9, no. 1 (2019): 3387, https://doi.org/10.1038/s41598-019-39350-8.

powerless and alone. I bet you see this all over your friend group and around your office!

The masculinization of women hasn't raised women's voices; it's silenced them. *The irony.* Everyday women who have labored under the rubric that women should act more like men to get ahead are so disconnected from their feminine that it's stunted their ability to ask for what they desire, and therefore it has retarded their ability to receive. If I had a dime for every woman who came to me absolutely confused about what it means to receive and how to ask the people in her life for what she needed, I'd be writing this book from the back seat of my Bentley. Yes, the problem is that bad, and chances are, it's why you made it this far into this book. This hampered ability to ask for what we desire—and receive it—has put otherwise intelligent women in a position of having to (at best) mime their needs to their men or (at worst) expect them to be mind readers. If we lack the ability to freely express our needs without worry about being considered weak or "crazy," how is that progress?

The idea that we don't need a man but we should *act like one* has trapped millions of women into a cycle of poor communication, frustration, and unreasonable, heartbreaking expectations that's left both men and women confused about how to even be together.

Femininity Has Taken a Beating on Multiple Fronts; Time for a Comeback

What I've shared in this chapter is meant to help you understand the historical, cultural, social, and economic influences that have come together to undermine our feminine nature as women in the United States. Under the guise of "moving us forward" (which you can now see means moving us away from our feminine), our connection to our feminine and our natural inclinations as women have been eroded. Not only were we duped into believing that all these advances were "progress" on all fronts, but the reality is, we've never worked harder or had to "prove" ourselves more in more aspects of our lives, while the relationships and families that were a significant source of the love and connectedness our feminine craves are flimsy impostors of what they once were. In the name of progress, we spend fewer hours each day with the people we love, we ship our babies off to daycare or to nannies, and the children we wanted so badly get two hours or less of our time daily,[60] *all so that we can one day have a "good" life.* Is that a model that honors the feminine? Is that the life the nurturer in you wants? Is that why you are working so hard to call in this baby?

What the history I have shared in this chapter demonstrates is how the process of masculinization of women was set in motion. You can see now how it has impacted our lives as women, how it has leeched a "be masculine to be successful" mentality into our minds, and how this disconnection from our feminine has hobbled us in our relationships and is leading to a life of frustration and despair. I know you want more. I will help you get there. But first, let's look at the data that shows in real terms why we have to bring the masculinization of women to a swift end in order to save ourselves...*and our fertility.*

60. *American Time Use Survey Summary - 2022 A01 Results*, U.S. Bureau of Labor Statistics, June 22, 2023, https://www.bls.gov/news.release/atus.nr0.htm.

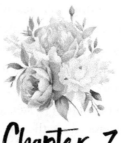

Chapter 7

The Feminine Isn't Frivolous; It's the Foundation of Our Families

The messaging by the 1970s was that women had "won." Exactly what we had won isn't clear, but as the initial fervor of the women's movement settled down, real women, living real lives outside the consequence-free echo chamber of academia, found themselves settling into an existence that was anything but the "feminist" utopia we had been so lavishly promised. The decades following proved to push women closer and closer to despair as we were dragged further away from our feminine nature. The data is consistent and heartbreaking—*girrrl, our overall quality of life has tanked.*

The Negative Impact of "Shifting Priorities"

The first place we see the most dramatic implications of the attack on femininity is in how it has destroyed our birth rate. While not everyone has wild dreams of driving around in a minivan full of screaming kids, the avalanche-like drop in birth rate since 1960 leads me to wonder how much longer carmakers are going to bother offering vehicles with a back seat! The longer the mainstreamed masculine messaging has endured, the further and faster the fertility rate has crashed—*and not recovered.*[1] Women in the United States have gone from having 3.443 babies each in 1960 to 1.784 in 2023.[2] That's insane. The population in the United States has steadily declined at a rapid pace and has not recovered since the Great Recession of 2008.[3] This has puzzled researchers; while there is typically a recovery in birth rate after a financial crisis, between 2007 and 2020, the drop in birth rate has been "dramatic."[4] At best, researchers have conservatively conjectured that this is a result of "shifting priorities."[5] The decline in birth rate also tracks with women having babies later, with the most highly educated women, meaning those who hold a master's degree or higher, not having their first babies until the median age of thirty.[6] That means they wait a full six years longer than their sisters who hold a high school diploma or less.[7]

Just because researchers aren't willing to make conclusions about the disastrous population data doesn't mean you can't, though. It's not an academic's job to tell you what to think. You can think for yourself. I bet your spidey senses were putting two and two together about why the birth rate is tanking at an alarming rate—particularly in light of the history and data I've shared in the last chapter. As an intelligent woman who prob-

1. "U.S. Fertility Rate 1950–2023."
2. "U.S. Fertility Rate 1950–2023."
3. Melissa S. Kearney, Phillip B. Levine, and Luke Pardue, "The Puzzle of Falling US Birth Rates since the Great Recession," *Journal of Economic Perspectives* 36, no. 1 (Winter 2022): 151–76, https://doi.org/10.1257/jep.36.1.151.
4. Kearney, Levine, and Pardue, "Falling US Birth Rates."
5. Kearney, Levine, and Pardue, "Falling US Birth Rates."
6. Gretchen Livingston, "For Most Highly Educated Women, Motherhood Doesn't Start Until the 30s," Pew Research Center, January 15, 2015, https://www.pewresearch.org/short-reads/2015/01/15/for-most-highly-educated-women-motherhood-doesnt-start-until-the-30s/.
7. Livingston, "Motherhood Doesn't Start."

isn't worried about her grants or cushy professorship being in jeopardy, I bet you can come to your own conclusions. You probably don't have to look further than your life and the lives of other women you know to see the connection between making work the priority and the drop in birth rate playing out. I'm sure you can see the price women have paid for burning the candle at both ends, chasing, proving, neglecting self-care, buying the scam of masculine achievement, putting off partnership until they've checked all the boxes, maybe holding themselves and their partners to crazy unreasonable standards, or consistently putting off baby-making for some imaginary "right" time.

Remember, none of this is about making you or your choices wrong. Nor am I saying there's only one definition of feminine. It's about awareness of the pattern of masculinization that has stunted our growth as women. How is it "progress" to basically shut down and devalue our innate nature as women? It isn't. But the consequences of our disconnection from the feminine aren't just seen in our individual lives; they have negatively impacted the lives of our children as well. If that doesn't get your attention as a mama in the making, I'm not sure what will.

We've Never Been More Unhappy

You'd think that, with all we had been promised since the 1960s, women would be happier today. We've never been more educated, wealthy, independent, or "free," nor have we had access to more choices that control the direction of our lives. There's virtually no pressure to get married or have babies other than whatever calling we have for either or both in our hearts. On the outside, all of these "advances" look like a massive win for the so-called women's movement. The problem is, despite all the trappings of victory, the win is, at best, a hollow one. Women in the United States are more unhappy today than they were prior to women's lib.[8] This means that we've worked our butts off based on masculine measures of success. Many of us struggle to have the babies we long for, and when we finally take a moment to look around our lives, far too many of us are asking, "*WTF?*"

This is shocking, but if we are honest, it's not altogether surprising. When you suppress nature for long enough, there is a reckoning, and it's rarely a pretty one. Mother Nature can be ruthless and exacting in her justice. What did we think would happen after decades of making our femininity wrong, suppressing our desires for love and family, and denying the calling of our highest selves? The artificial, masculine super-woman propped up by an anti-feminine media, education system, and political "elite" has fallen flat. The data proves it, and more women are waking up to the lie.

A study done by Betsey Stevenson and Justin Wolfers found that, according to measures of subjective well-being, women's happiness declined "both absolutely and relative to men" during the period from 1972 to 2006.[9] This decline is "found across various datasets" and "is pervasive across demographic groups and industrialized countries."[10] If you are wondering what the definition of "subjective well-being" is, researchers used the following question to measure it: "Taken all together, how would you say things are these days...would you say that you are very happy, pretty happy, or not too happy?" In the study, researchers looked at aspects of life such as marriage, health, finances, and their work.[11] To be clear, they didn't just

8. Betsey Stevenson and Justin Wolfers, "The Paradox of Declining Female Happiness" (working paper, National Bureau of Economic Research, Cambridge, Massachusetts, 2009), https://www.nber.org/papers/w14969.

9. Stevenson and Wolfers, "Paradox of Declining Female Happiness."

10. Stevenson and Wolfers, "Paradox of Declining Female Happiness."

11. Stevenson and Wolfers, "Paradox of Declining Female Happiness."

use one-off data to draw their conclusions. They relied upon the General Social Survey (GSS), which has been used in the United States since 1972.[12]

Women in the 1970s reported higher subjective well-being than men, but over the decades, a new gender gap emerged— *men reporting a higher level of happiness than women!*[13] What's even more interesting is that women of all education groups have become less happy over time, with declines in happiness being the most dramatic among the college-educated.[14] *Whoops!* Weren't education, the jobs that come as a result, and freedom from the albatross of the home supposed to make us happier and free? Remember all the claims and promises made by the women's movement? *Yoo-hoo!* We were promised more education, more money, more freedom—where's that utopia? Looks like we succeeded in getting all the "mores," yet with fewer traditional feminine measures of success found through love, relationships, and family, women today are unfulfilled and miserable. Sorry, Mamas. *We got played.*

This decline in happiness was also found to impact young girls during the same period; young girls faced a steep decline relative to boys, which was even more marked than that in adults.[15]

According to researchers, the decline in women's happiness can't be blown off as just a natural decline after the initial fervor and excitement of the women's movement.[16] The tentacles of this significant drop in happiness are impacting women's happiness in our homes—both in our marriages and in our overall satisfaction with our home lives.[17] Having analyzed this

---

12. Stevenson and Wolfers, "Paradox of Declining Female Happiness."
13. Stevenson and Wolfers, "Paradox of Declining Female Happiness."
14. Stevenson and Wolfers, "Paradox of Declining Female Happiness."
15. Stevenson and Wolfers, "Paradox of Declining Female Happiness."
16. Stevenson and Wolfers, "Paradox of Declining Female Happiness."
17. Stevenson and Wolfers, "Paradox of Declining Female Happiness."

thirty-five years of data, researchers concluded that these patterns of declining happiness may be an indication of changing realities for women in that life satisfaction used to mean "satisfaction at home," but now it includes "satisfaction at work" and navigating dramatic changes in societal norms.[18] Women are trying to achieve satisfaction in multiple aspects of their lives while faced with increased single parenthood, increased divorce, and decreased pressure on men to commit and support their children if a woman gets pregnant (thanks to birth control and abortion), and doing so under those changing circumstances is proving difficult.[19]

While Stevenson and Wolford were reluctant to make any definitive conclusions and don't exactly call out the women's movement for the sham the data proves it to be, at least according to women's overall subjective well-being, you are a smart cookie. I know that based on your own experience and the honest experiences of women, you can see for yourself that our reality as women today is hardly what we were led to believe it would be, and we are paying for it with our happiness.[20]

Another study observed that women in their sixties have some of the highest rates of antidepressant use—and the trend continues upward.[21] Arguably, women at that stage in their lives would be cruising, happy, reaping the spoils of their education, wealth, and boundless choices, but with this level of antidepressant use, the picture isn't so rosy.[22]

18. Stevenson and Wolfers, "Paradox of Declining Female Happiness."
19. Stevenson and Wolfers, "Paradox of Declining Female Happiness."
20. Stevenson and Wolfers, "Paradox of Declining Female Happiness."
21. Debra J. Brody and Qiuping Gu, *Antidepressant Use Among Adults: United States, 2015-2018*, Centers for Disease Control and Prevention, September 2020, https://www.cdc.gov/nchs/products/databriefs/db377.htm.
22. Brody and Gu, *Antidepressant Use Among Adults*.

"Old Fashioned" Women Are Happier

As much as it may cause some of those reading this book to retch when I say it, the facts don't lie: women who hold on to more traditional structures in their lives, such as marriage, having babies, and cultivating a joyous home life are, well, *happier*.

As noted earlier, the General Social Survey has been collecting data on overall happiness in adults in the United States since 1972.[23] Based on that data, it's been reported that married people are a whopping thirty percentage points more happy than the unmarried.[24] Researchers controlled for variances such as education, wealth, and race, and the findings survived controls for such differences.[25] It's notable that happier people tend to get married and be in committed relationships, so higher levels of happiness should be expected in married people, even if the marriage in and of itself did not singularly add to each person's overall happiness.[26] In an age where most people just read headlines and mistake them for facts, it's important to note that fairly recently, there was a viral claim that married women were less happy, but like much of the noise running around the internet, *that claim is absolute fiction.*[27]

It also appears that, for American women, the road to

23. Sam Peltzman, "The Socio Political Demography of Happiness" (working paper, George J. Stigler Center for the Study of the Economy & the State), http://dx.doi.org/10.2139/ssrn.4508123.

24. Peltzman, "Demography of Happiness."

25. Peltzman, "Demography of Happiness."

26. Iskra Fileva, "Is Marriage a Bad Deal for Women?," Psychology Today, May 16, 2021, https://www.psychologytoday.com/us/blog/the-philosophers-diaries/202105/is-marriage-a-bad-deal-for-women.

27. Kelsey Piper, "A New Book Says Married Women Are Miserable. Don't Believe It," Vox, June 4, 2019, https://www.vox.com/future-perfect/2019/6/4/18650969/married-women-miserable-fake-paul-dolan-happiness.

happiness runs *through* married motherhood, not away from it.[28] In 2020, 69% of mothers ages eighteen to fifty-five were completely or somewhat satisfied with their lives, compared with 61% of childless women the same age.[29] There was a dip in women's happiness between 2019 and 2020 when COVID set in, but the dip was bigger for childless women.[30] As discussed in previous sections, it's obvious that we as women still want significant elements of what's often dismissed as "traditional" lives because, despite having careers, we still want babies, still seek marriage (or at least long-term committed partnerships), and still desire happy homes, even if we start the process of family-building "later" or start alone. As much as second-wave "feminism" paraded the banner of breaking free from the oppression of the family, it turns out that *women still crave it.* Women and children are both better off financially and experientially when families are based in married or long-term partnerships.[31] Certainly, this presumes a happy marriage or partnership, *but why would we presume otherwise, considering the wide latitude of choices we as women have today?* While some may try to defeat this reality by arguing in terms of extremes, you can't get around the fact that the wedding and fertility indus-

---

28. Brad Wilcox and Wendy Wang, "The Married-Mom Advantage," *Atlantic*, December 27, 2022, https://www.theatlantic.com/ideas/archive/2022/12/motherhood-marriage-pandemic-covid-children/672563/.

29. Wilcox and Wang, "Married-Mom Advantage."

30. Wilcox and Wang, "Married-Mom Advantage."

31. Kay S. Hymowitz, "The Indispensable Institution," *City Journal*, September 15, 2023, https://www.city-journal.org/article/review-of-the-two-parent-privilege-by-melissa-kearney, discussing Melissa Kearney, *The Two-Parent Privilege: How Americans Stopped Getting Married and Started Falling Behind* (Chicago, IL: University of Chicago Press, 2023).

tries are $70 billion[32] and $8.1 billion[33] powerhouses in the United States, with women leading the charge when it comes to spending on both. So much for educating babies, family, and marriage out of a woman's heart. One needn't look further than someone's spending to see what they value most.

All this data lines up with what I see in my own coaching practice. While I by no means pass judgment on how women structure or choose to build their families, it's clear from my own observations that women who seek to have babies within marriages and long-term partnerships are dramatically happier and have more overall support—financial and emotional— than those pursuing motherhood on their own. Even those who are pursuing single motherhood by choice admit that their goal is to one day have a partner and get married. The women I work with, despite their advanced education, incredible professional accomplishments, and even celebrity, all share, in one way or another, that their careers alone don't provide the fulfillment that they ultimately desire. They want love, babies, and to come home at the end of the day to a happy family. The funny thing is, not one of them has ever expressed feeling oppressed or hampered in their life because of those beautifully basic-in-the-best-way-possible desires.

Live the Masculine Dream, Then Struggle to Have a Baby— Whoops!

Let's say, like me, you bought into the propaganda that said

---

32. Abha Bhattarai, "Smaller Cakes, Shorter Dresses, Bigger Diamonds: The Pandemic Is Shaking Up the $73 Billion Wedding Industry," *Washington Post*, February 11, 2021, https://www.washingtonpost.com/road-to-recovery/2021/02/11/zoom-weddings-covid-diamond-rings/.

33. *Fertility Clinics in the US - Market Size (2004–2029)*, IBISWorld Industry Reports, November 15, 2023, https://www.ibisworld.com/industry-statistics/market-size/fertility-clinics-united-states/.

motherhood is the lesser choice and the only way to be truly liberated was to outwork, out-achieve, and out-earn your own mother so you'd never have to depend on a man like she did or be disappointed by one like she was. Harsh, I know, but follow me on this. This means you busted your butt through undergrad and plowed your way through a master's degree, law school, medical school, or whatever professional training you've had with the iron will of a woman who was damned sure she'd never let anyone oppress her. Your grades were as enviable as your work ethic, and everybody—I mean everybody—knows you get the job done. Then *boom!* You look up from your work to discover you're in your mid-ish to late thirties, the workhorse machine schtick has run its course, and it's time to start paying attention to the pang in your heart. You wanna be a mama. *Insert film noir plot twist music.*

The problem is that the moment you step into the baby-making ring, you're slapped with scary statistics about how difficult it is to get pregnant "at your age." The do-the-smart-thing rule-follower in you is going, "But, wait! I did all the things I was supposed to, and now you're telling me it's too late to have the one thing I realize I want more than anything? Are you f*cking kidding me?!" When this happens, many women feel confused or even betrayed. Think about all the discipline you've exercised and the hard work you've done to this point to not "ruin your life" by having a baby "too young" or with the "wrong partner." You played your cards perfectly under the masculine paradigm, only to be hit with scary statistics and long-faced lectures about how you "waited too long" and your options are limited. I know I felt angry about this kind of treatment, and so have the overwhelming majority of my clients. It's like being told to finish every last bit of your dinner *before you can even think of having dessert*, then having that dessert yanked away after all of your patience and discipline. That's the irony of the scam we've been sold. *You can do absolutely anything with* *no judgment or limitations, as long as it's not baby-making.* Can you imagine the fervor that would be kicked up if you walked in for a job interview and were immediately told you had very little chance of job success because you were too old? Just imagine the pitchforks, torches, and news helicopters buzzing around the place! "You're too old to have a baby," though? Not so much.

Women who want to have babies "later in life" face way more scrutiny and judgment than some dude who up and decides one day he wants to hack off his genitals and start calling himself Barbee. I promise you, that guy would get boatloads of compassion and support, while biological women who are equally following their hearts get a condescending, stern-faced lecture. How's that for a double standard? Men who reject their biology are elevated, celebrated, and accommodated, while women embracing theirs get slapped with stats. To add insult to injury, the same "feminists" who side-eye you for being a "breeder" will welcome old Barbee with open arms. *Oh, the masculine matriarchy!*

You did exactly what you were told would make you a happy, productive, unoppressed member of society, only to find yourself in a spiral of regret and self-loathing, wondering if you wasted your precious childbearing years doing what you thought of as the right thing, only to find it wasn't—or at least, not exactly. Then, like clockwork, you're yanked back into your masculine energy, punishing yourself for not knowing what was actively being kept from you, and trying harder. As I said earlier, the game was rigged, Mama and you, like me, got scammed. You have credentials out the wazoo, you're gainfully employed, so you can support your kids, and you've never been more ready, but you're being told it's too late. *Gulp.*

Professional women got hit hardest by the scam. Census data shows us that within the scary population decline in the United States, highly educated women are creating a "delayer boom," which means that our segment of the population is waiting much later to have babies, *but we are still having fewer babies* than women with less education.[34] We also know that babies born after assisted conception are more likely to be born to mothers of a higher socioeconomic status.[35] Research points to social factors such as educational attainment, labor force participation, and marriage delays for why women are having babies later—without asking the more pointed questions about how women got "there" and if "there" is a good thing for the women and our society.[36] But doing something naughty, like asking such a dangerously-disruptive-to-the-masculinization-narrative question, would further expose the scam. *We certainly don't want to do that!* Who'd want to wake millions of women up to the idea that they'd been had and that they are powerful, worthy, and awesome exactly as they are, femininity and all?

While women are having babies later, we are having fewer and are possibly not living our baby-making dreams to the fullest based on our age, remaining fertile years, and the brow-beating we get for being "late to the game."[37] When you consider the enormity of this and how many women may have given up on their dreams because they were shamed and made to feel ridiculous, it's heartbreaking.

---

34. "Census Bureau Reports 'Delayer Boom' as More Educated Women Have Children Later," United States Census Bureau, May 9, 2011, https://www.census.gov/newsroom/releases/archives/fertility/cb11-83.html.

35. Rachel Imrie et al., "Socioeconomic Status and Fertility Treatment Outcomes in High-income Countries: A Review of the Current Literature," *Human Fertility* 26, no. 1 (2023): 27–37, https://doi.org/10.1080/14647273.2021.1957503.

36. Gretchen Livingston, "They're Waiting Longer, but U.S. Women Today More Likely to Have Children than a Decade Ago," Pew Research Center, January 18, 2018, https://www.pewresearch.org/social-trends/2018/01/18/theyre-waiting-longer-but-u-s-women-today-more-likely-to-have-children-than-a-decade-ago/.

37. "Delayer Boom."

Living in a Masculine State of Chronic Stress Makes It Harder to Conceive

I remember being told on numerous occasions by my allopathic physicians that stress had absolutely nothing to do with my fertility issues. I was told that there was no evidence to support that claim and that if I just "trusted the science" and jammed myself full of the drugs Big Pharma was all too happy to sell me, I could magically override my insane lifestyle as a prosecutor and the chronic stress I was under. Even though that seemed crazy to me, I thought to myself, "I went to law school, not medical school—what do I know?" I have so much compassion for the version of me that abdicated her authority and didn't listen to her gut. My gut was right, and not listening to her cost me dearly. Funny how feminine intuition is *still* so easily dismissed as hysterics sixty years after the women's movement promised us better.

Chances are, when it comes to your questions about stress and fertility, you've probably been blown off by at least one eye-rolling doctor too. You are about to be vindicated, Mama. Real data is showing us that, indeed, stress is detrimental to your fertility. A study published in 2014 found that higher levels of stress, as measured by salivary alpha-amylase, are associated with a longer time to pregnancy and an increased risk of infertility.[38] Researchers also found that women in the highest quartile of alpha-amylase levels at baseline were twice as likely to subsequently experience infertility.[39] There was another study

38. Courtney Denning-Johnson Lynch et al., "Preconception Stress Increases the Risk of Infertility: Results from a Couple-Based Prospective Cohort Study—The LIFE Study," *Human Reproduction* (Oxford, England) 29, no. 5 (2014), 1067–75, https://doi.org/10.1093/humrep/deu032.
39. Kristin L. Rooney and Alice D. Domar, "The Relationship between Stress and Infertility," *Dialogues in Clinical Neuroscience* 20, no. 1 (2018), 41–47. https://doi.org/10.31887/DCNS.2018.20.1/klrooney.

in 2016, based on 135 IVF patients, where cortisol (which indicates stress!) was measured through samplings of hair, which helps measure cortisol for longer periods of time (three to six months). The higher the cortisol level, the worse the pregnancy rate.[40]

These findings confirm what most fertility patients believe: psychological symptoms of stress negatively impact fertility.[41] You don't have to be a scientist to know that chronic stress is terrible for your health. Everyone knows it causes disease, and when in a cortisol-laden fight-or-flight mode, the body reprioritizes energy away from nonessential functions (like fertility) to respond to the stressor.[42] Today, the primary source of our stress is self-imposed. We aren't being chased by saber-toothed tigers anymore. The demands of daily life as success-oriented women can keep us on the hamster wheel of fight or flight. Just imagine the impact of being stuck in that state for five to ten years, particularly when we've learned to attach our self-worth to a masculine measure of success. *Holy Moses!*

Do women get pregnant when they are stressed? Of course —it happens all the time—but fertility may not be an issue for those women, and they may not be at the level of success you are. The smarter inquiry is whether the stress is negatively impacting *you*, and I think you know the answer. The bottom line here is that there are increasing amounts of evidence (the White Coats are just finally acknowledging it) that stress has a negative impact on fertility, and sustained stress is likely making it worse.[43] The good news is that interventions that support women as they struggle with fertility are associated

40. Rooney and Domar, "Relationship between Stress and Infertility."
41. Rooney and Domar, "Relationship between Stress and Infertility."
42. "What Happens to Your Body During the Fight-or-Flight Response?," Cleveland Clinic, December 8, 2019, https://health.clevelandclinic.org/what-happens-to-your-body-during-the-fight-or-flight-response.
43. Rooney and Domar, "Relationship between Stress and Infertility."

with decreases in depression and increases in pregnancy rates.[44] I see the truth of this play out in my coaching programs and the incredible corresponding success of my clients.

It's about time "science" finally caught up with what fertility patients know from the trenches. Having lived this journey myself and having coached and taught thousands of high-achieving professional women from around the world as they try to have babies, I can tell you firsthand that chronic stress is sabotaging the fertility of professional women. Not only do we wait longer to have babies, but by the time we get around to it, we have decades of crushing stress trapped in our bodies, and we pay the price for living in the masculine matrix *with our fertility*.

It's unnatural and absurd to think that women could sustain stress like men and face no biological consequences. Women are not men. Men don't have babies. We are equal but not the same. That should be obvious, but we are living in the aftermath of the warped cultural conditioning that's spent decades propagandizing otherwise. The insane success stories found in my own coaching practice are proof positive of what I'm saying here. When my ladies stop acting like men, they start having babies. This is true regardless of age and how many times they've failed with treatment in the past. In fact, some even do the thing White Coats say isn't possible "at their age" and with their "conditions": *they get pregnant naturally*.

Coincidence? Causation? Correlation?

Stress is a critical factor in the overall decline in fertility in the United States. While indeed there are other contributing factors, I believe that at a foundational level, the most devastating attack has been programming femininity out of women

---

44. Rooney and Domar, "Relationship between Stress and Infertility."

in the name of "progress." Self-care, restoration, nurturing, and being versus doing are values women have had to subordinate in order to "get ahead." They also happen to be things that can help mitigate the stress and overwhelm that are an epidemic for women in America. Holding women to a masculine standard isn't lifting them up; it's breaking them down by denying biological and spiritual realities that make women the beautiful and unique beings we are.

The decline in fertility rates directly corresponds with the rise in the women's movement and the sexual revolution.[45] It's undeniable. Is this just an unfortunate coincidence? Were these movements the sole cause of the decline in our fertility? I don't believe in coincidence, and it would be intellectually dishonest to say that these two movements combined are the *sole* reason for the perilous decline in American fertility. However, when you combine these movements with the rise of chemical birth control, selling women the idea that a career outside the home is "progress," no-fault divorce, and the promise of having it all (and doing it all), you can see how we got here. The shockwave of these movements produced a decades-long, fundamental shift for women in American society, where the "feminine mystique" was traded for a masculine ideal that has left the female "beneficiaries" of these movements having fewer babies, struggling to have them when they do, and more unhappy than ever.

Time for a Feminine Homecoming

Getting scammed sucks, but the upside is that when you find out about the scam and how big it was, you aren't likely to let it happen again. We've blown the lid off the big fat lie we were told about the feminine. We can now see, plain as day, data in

---

45. "U.S. Fertility Rate 1950–2023."

hand, that there are serious consequences that women and American families have suffered as a result of being scammed out of our feminine nature. The crazy part is, as I've said, we were sold the idea that subordinating (or even obliterating) our femininity for a masculine paradigm was progress and was "advancing" us as women. We were supposed to be better off working long hours, acting like men, competing with men, never asking for help, abandoning our self-care, and betraying every instinct we had to rest, cry, or shout that *something is wrong.* It was supposed to be the "smart" and "responsible" thing to do to wait to try for a baby, but when the "right" time rolls around, we are practically begging our ovaries to toss us one good egg, for f*ck's sake. Those days are over. It's time that we, as women, reclaim our femininity and rewrite the rules of success in a way that honors our femininity instead of marginalizing it. Our happiness and our families depend on it.

You're awake now, Mama. You've been pink-pilled. You have information upon which to make a different, feminine choice. The question becomes…will you?

In the next chapter, we're going to talk about making space for the feminine in your life and what that might look like. I know it sounds strange that we as women need to learn to consider the feminine again, but based on what you've read so far, clearly, we do. The exciting part is that this isn't a one-size-fits-all proposition. We fell for that once with the "masculine is more" narrative we've been laboring under for decades. What I'm going to map out for you in the next couple of chapters is feminine in its operation and in its execution. How's that for a breath of feminine fresh air?

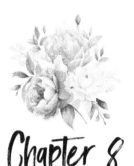

Chapter 8
Finding Space for Feminine First

A t this point in our journey together, you are beginning to understand what the feminine is, her interplay with the masculine, and how we've gotten scammed out of her warm presence in our lives. You are now familiar with how her absence has negatively impacted our lives, wrecked our relationships, destabilized our families, and can negatively impact our fertility. Our disconnectedness from our femininity impacts us emotionally, spiritually, and biologically. If we make the support we desire wrong, if we can't ask for what we need, if our relationships are strained and lacking, and we aren't consistently investing in restorative self-care, how could we possibly be open to receive and therefore conceive?

You can see the impact of the masculine paradigm playing out in your life right now and on your journey. Based on everything you've learned up to this point, the value and role of your feminine should no longer be the subject of any reasonable dispute. Our work now is to consciously cultivate exactly *where* you want to discover and reconnect with her in your life.

Let's start off by understanding that the goal here isn't a pendulum swing into living your life entirely from the feminine. That would be just as lame as being 100% in your masculine. Remember what I said in chapter 3: it's about finesse and marshaling these two energies within you. The masculine needs the softness of the feminine, and the feminine needs the structure and execution offered by the masculine. If you were hanging out in your feminine all day every day, life would be a lot less organized, deadlines would get missed, and you'd meander in your life pondering questions and possibly never doing what it took to get answers! *Who wants that?* You already know how fried you are from living in Man Mode masculine. Let's be done with the masculine that drives extremes, shall we? Can you see why allowing the masculine and feminine to work together is so important? That's why I call the principle I'm sharing here Feminine First. The goal isn't feminine *only*, just first.

The Principle of Feminine First

Feminine First means choosing to be *led* by your creative, curious, spiritual, intuitive, nurturing, sensual, and loving self first, then allowing your masculine side to execute on your Feminine First desires. You have already proven that you can execute and follow through. Just look at the success you have built in your life! What makes the Feminine First approach different is its starting point is your feminine, aka your heart, your intuition, your desires. You check in with those aspects of yourself first, then and only then, do you let your head kick in. Remember, one more time for the seats in the back, that none of this is about making your masculine "bad" or a "lesser" resource within you. We are simply shifting who is in the driver's seat. The point is to find a mix of the masculine and feminine that works for you and honors the uniqueness of your quirks and values.

To really drive the principle of Feminine First home for you, I will share a powerful question I use to not only engage my feminine, but to check whether I am living by Feminine First: *What would the creative, curious, spiritual, intuitive, nurturing, sensual, and loving side of me do or say about this?* Rather than reacting and going back into my boring, default masculine patterns, I call upon my feminine with that question. I consciously choose to consider my Feminine First. If you are anything like me, you know exactly what your masculine would have you do. We are engaging a different set up muscles with the feminine, and it will feel a bit awkward at first. That's okay. I also want to point out that each of the seven feminine characteristics I refer to earlier in this paragraph (i.e., creative, curious, spiritual) are different, and they might each have something different to say. Great! But don't worry. You don't have to answer the question seven times to engage each aspect of you. Simply ask the question *once* and listen. They may all chime in or not. One may speak louder than others. That's cool too. Listen and learn. Don't overthink this—*that would be your masculine hijacking the process.*

As you play with the principle of Feminine First, I want you to understand that you can't do this "wrong." Leading from your feminine is an exploration. As I said back in chapter 3, the expression of your feminine will be personal to you, like a fingerprint. You get to have fun with Feminine First. Let your feminine unfold and reveal herself to you.

Where Are You Most in Need of Feminine First?

You have the masculine nailed, so under the principle of Feminine First, the idea is to bring more elements of the feminine into your life, and that consideration starts with taking a survey of your life as you live it now. *Where, instinctively, based on what you've read here and how you currently feel about your life, do you know you want to live Feminine First?*

I know that by now you might be screaming, *"Everywhere!"* So let's break this inquiry down into segments.

Do you know what you really want? I mean *really* want. I know that's a massive question to ask, but sh*t, if I don't ask it, after upending your apple cart about masculinized success and exposing how you've been robbed of an essential part of yourself and have been living a misogynist lie, who the hell will? If you leaned into your feminine, what would she tell you about what you really, really want?

I don't expect you to be able to answer this question fully right now, and chances are, after you begin considering aspects of your life where you want to live more Feminine First, your desires will evolve. Asking this question now will give you the chance to consider it in the background as you think about where you want to apply Feminine First in your life.

Let's get specific. Do you want to approach your work with a more Feminine First perspective? I know you know how to grind and outwork everyone around you; does that still work for you? Does that line up with what you desire in your life? Do you truly want to keep doing what you do? Is there a secret, slightly scary part of you that just wants to quit, start a sustainable farm, and raise your babies with their bare feet in the dirt as you lead sound healing retreats and let your man do manlike things like bringing home the bacon? There's no shame in that game, Mama! Even if a farm with chickens and goats doesn't sound awesome to you, I bet you get the picture. If you think of work from a Feminine First perspective, what would you choose for work? Remember, it's okay to play here. Don't worry about the how. Your masculine will figure that part out.

What about your relationship? How would you approach it from Feminine First? How might things be different between you and your partner if you brought the *creative, curious, spiritual, intuitive, nurturing, sensual, and loving side* of you to the forefront? Would your communication with your man be different? Would you be more open to receiving from him? I tell my ladies all the time that if they approach their man the way a man would, he will treat them like a man! Makes sense, right? If you started showing up Feminine First with your man, what might change?

Now, if you are not currently partnered, how might Feminine First change the way you approach the possibility of new relationships? Might you have considered relationships differently in the past if you were looking through the lens of the feminine? If you are planning to be a single mother by choice, how might you pursue that in a Feminine First way? There are no right answers here—we've thrown masculinization out the window. The most important thing is to discover your answers from the perspective of Feminine First.

Looking at what you want, your work, and your relationship from a Feminine First perspective is a powerful setup for bringing more of the feminine to your fertility journey. Think about it: your desires, your work, and your relationship are top of mind all the time. If you start considering those things from Feminine First, you make the transition to thinking that way when it comes to your fertility natural and, dare I say, more graceful. When you get clear on what you want and consistently ask what *the creative, curious, spiritual, intuitive, nurturing, sensual, and loving side* of you thinks, and begin taking different action in your life as a result, you can't help but reduce your stress, make confident decisions you love, and dramatically improve your relationships. In the end, you feel more peace, calm, and confidence when you engage the principle of Feminine First.

Let's now talk about how this can start to look on your fertility journey.

A Fertility Journey Informed by the Feminine?

If you've been super masculine in your approach to conceiving, how would you shift to approach it informed by your femininity? What does the *creative, curious, spiritual, intuitive, nurturing, sensual, and loving side of you* say about how you want to go about TTC from here on out? Is your feminine super excited about back-to-back IVF cycles for a year? Is she harboring a secret dream to conceive this baby naturally? You certainly wouldn't be the first woman who was bullied into IVF but later followed her heart and got pregnant naturally. I'm not in any way saying one is better than the other—natural or the use of reproductive technology. They both rock! Maybe you are actually longing to move into IVF after trying naturally for years because something in your heart tells you that you need additional support. The point is for you to follow your heart and trust yourself when it comes to where you'd like to have Feminine First show up on your journey.

Let's talk about what your feminine says about your relationship and this journey. Do you want your man to play a more supportive role? Does he need to know how scared and stressed you've been? Perhaps it's time to drop the stiff upper lip and give him the chance to be there for you. Your feminine likely has a whole lot to say about how she thinks things in your relationship could be different as you live this journey. When it comes to relationships, as you saw in earlier chapters, the masculine can mess with our heads and disconnect us from our partners by making us think vulnerability or wanting support is weakness. Chances are, your feminine is going to invite you to show your partner what's real for you. Trust her.

Remember, our femininity is about options, creative, heart-based solutions, based on the vision we have for our lives. Our feminine is trusting and has faith when our masculine doesn't. Are there things you've been longing to do on your fertility journey, but have been afraid to? Check in with your feminine. She's been on mute for a while; chances are, she has a lot to say.

There's No Blowup, Just a Level Up

Deciding where you want to bring more feminine into your life and on this journey isn't about making your previous way of being wrong, blowing up your life, or being so far gone it's too late to have your babies. Going to those extreme conclusions is just another form of the masculine matrix keeping you trapped in the lie. I've helped a fifty-two-year-old woman have her miracle baby after she woke up to the masculine lies in her life. Today, she's living her dream with her precious baby on her hip, happy as a clam, while most people are zombie-ing their way into lackluster retirement! Her feminine told her that her baby-making days weren't over, and—funny thing—her feminine was right!

Look around your life and consider where it could use more feminine awesomeness. The questions I asked you to explore will help you build out some ideas of how that might look. At its core, Feminine First is about reclaiming your peace by living in whole truth; no more shushing the feminine.

Now that you know where you want more of your feminine in your life and are getting a better sense of what that might look like, let's talk about what it takes to reclaim her so you can have more of her goodness.

Chapter 9

The Fearless Feminine: Unleash Her Now—It's Not Too Late

I know this has been a lot to take in, and you are quite possibly exhausted. The good news is, we are going to get into some super cool sh*t. I want to make it clear though that, in light of what you've learned, you may find yourself oscillating between anger, disbelief, and maybe even wanting to reject this outright—even with all the data I've provided. At the end of the day, though, the truth of what I've shared remains. We see it playing out in American society right now. It's crippled generations and weakened us as people. Deep down, you know what I have shared here is true—we have been scammed out of our feminine. And hey, if it makes you feel better, don't forget to check out the sources I list in my endnotes. The feminine is curious by nature, so if you feel called, let my sources be a springboard for your own research and continued edification.

Awakening in our context here is about becoming aware of the lies we're told about femininity, motherhood, success, men, relationships, and our innate power as women. Just imagine what's possible for you when, rather than being led down one narrow hallway of half-truths, the walls get busted down, and there's possibility as far as the eye can see. Awakening isn't easy, but it's awesome.

Now, chances are, you're wondering how the hell to discover and reclaim the femininity hidden from you by a system that told you it was weak, masculinized your approach to life, propagandized homemaking and having babies as the ignorantly pitiful choice, and made you think you had to hide this beautiful part of you from your man. As always, I've gotchu, Boo. I'm going to share some ideas that helped me snatch my life back from the clutches of the masculine matrix. Don't worry, it can be done. It may feel like a huge undertaking amid your fertility journey, but I assure you, there's never been a better time to do it, nor a better context in which to do it. I consistently see women who are facing less than 10% chances of conceiving unleash their feminine using my methodology, and boom, baby! That fact alone should get your engines revving—and if you doubt it, go watch a few interviews with my amazing clients on YouTube. The proof is in the pregnant-mama-making pudding.

Reclaiming the Feminine—Your Granddaughters Will Thank You

You should also be aware that the reclamation of your femininity isn't just about or for you. It's for your children, grandchildren, and generations of women you will never meet. I know that sounds lofty, but it's real, and it's one of the greatest gifts you can give humanity. Seeing the destruction of the family, the unhappiness of women today, the horrific decline in our population, the epidemic of fertility issues that plague us, and the pale, weak, confused, and overmedicated people we have become, you have a chance to be a leader, an example. The changes in attitude and behavior I will share here will help you see yourself differently, and in turn, you will see those around you—and the world in general—with new eyes. It's pretty f*cking exciting.

A word of caution as we get started: chose one focus area at a time. It took decades of masculine programming to get you off the feminine track, so it's going to take a minute for you to get back on. That doesn't mean it will take forever, but what I know from personal experience is that if you take one focus area at a time and give it your undivided attention, you can onboard the feminine more quickly and sustainably, then move on to the next. I also encourage you to move through the focus areas in the order they're presented here. You are a grown woman, so ultimately do as you wish, but I like to start with a strong foundation, and therefore I present the methodology in this way.

Feminine, Are We in a Relationship?

The first step in any reclamation—or in some cases *discovery*—of your feminine begins with creating your own unique relationship with her. I know that if you haven't had much of a relationship with your feminine since early childhood, you might be thinking, "Where do I even start?" The place to start is by identifying the beliefs you currently hold about femininity in general. Said another way, when you think about femininity, what thoughts come to mind? There's no right answer here. The point is to understand where you stand with your feminine today, not what you aspire for her to be. Maybe you think she's weak? Perhaps you think she's all about pink, frilly things with sparkles? It's possible you believe feminine women can't be taken seriously. You might also think femininity is unsafe. Whatever the case may be, do yourself a solid by being brutally honest. Don't beat yourself up if you find out you distrust or even hate your feminine. There's no judgment here. The point is to get to the truth so you can find your way back to her.

Believe it or not, she has always been there for you, and she's waiting with open arms.

Once you know where your relationship with your feminine stands, you can reclaim that relationship by deciding what it will be from here on out. It's the stuff of true feminine leadership to carefully consider, from a place of love, curiosity, and openness, how you choose to interact with this part of yourself. The masculine matrix taught you to suppress and disregard your feminine, so how will you be with her now? Because the feminine is the part of you who is creative, spiritual, intuitive, nurturing, and sensual, who sits with questions rather than demanding immediate answers, and who is concerned with being, not doing, you've got some territory to cover, Mama. The good news is that it's fun territory! What kind of relationship do you want to have with these aspects of yourself?

To get you thinking and, dare I say, *feeling* (the feeling part of you is feminine!) through this process, here are some questions to consider in the context of what your relationship with your feminine will be:

- Will you listen when she tells you something isn't right?
- Will you take the nap she's nudging you to take?
- Will you say *yes* to things she desires and *no* to things she hates?
- Will you take the art class she's been dying to take?
- Will you ditch your drab clothing for something that feels glorious on your skin?
- Will you move your body when she tells you to dance?
- Will you honor her by telling those around you the truth?
- Will you start taking better care of yourself?

- Will you tell your partner what you really need, with love, patience, and expectation?
- Will you let her guide you to a relationship with GUS?
- Will you let her guide you to a circle of like-minded women to call your sisterhood?
- Will you trust the desire she's placed in your heart to be a mom, knowing your baby is on the way?

You don't need to have answers to all these questions now. Let them whet your appetite for what's possible through a relationship with your feminine. Consider what these questions show you is possible when you consciously cultivate a relationship with your feminine. Rest? Truth? Freedom? Love? Connection? Trust? When you allow your feminine to meaningfully come back into your life, the sky's the limit, baby. Also, take note of which questions got you most excited! That's a powerful indicator from your feminine of what she desires most.

Lastly, as you begin to reclaim your relationship with your feminine, remember the word of caution I gave you earlier. It's easy to go into blame and regret here, when we consider how disconnected from our whole selves we've been. I've been there, and I can tell you it's a waste of your energy. Just know, those feelings are your masculine trying to reassert its dominance and keep you "safe" by going back to what you know— even if what you know kind of sucks. Make the conscious decision to keep your eyes up and forward-focused. We can't change the past, but this is your chance to pivot. No pity parties —just pivot.

No Demonizing the Masculine

There is a strong temptation when we do this work to get angry and want to blame or demonize all things masculine. Be mindful of this. A hallmark of that trap is to be temporarily blinded to the masculine's value and purpose. Don't do that. Reclaiming and crafting a relationship of our own design with the feminine doesn't require us to make the masculine wrong in any way. Seeking to demonize the masculine side of yourself is more of the masculine matrix death rattle seeking to keep you locked in a cycle of misery. The power of feminine influence on our thinking is the acknowledgment of the fact that multiple things can be true at the same time. You can be happy and sad. You can have desires and be grateful. We are multifaceted beings, and the need to make everything black and white with no subtlety is just another lie. The need to polarize is just more propaganda. You can have a strong relationship with your feminine while marshaling her with your masculine so you can be productive and powerful in your vision and purpose. Women who are truly successful on this journey and in their lives become masterful at knowing when to turn down their masculine and turn up their feminine, and they have sincere appreciation for the value of both.

Righteous and Radical Receiving

Want to flex feminine in a gorgeously glorious way? Receive. As women, we are physically and metaphorically receivers. My ladies hear me shouting this all the time on my podcast and in my programs: *conceiving is all about receiving.* In the decade-plus that I have been coaching women to fertility success, I have seen that the ability to receive is the place within our femininity where we are most stunted. The masculine matrix has placed so much judgment, shame, and heaviness on receiving that women have gotten terrible at it. For the sake of clarity, I will define *receiving* for you here in the same way that I have in the past:

The ability to accept love, time, money, gifts, favors, attention, support, blessings, acts of kindness, compliments, privileges, and priority without shame, guilt, condition, or the requirement of immediate and equal reciprocity.

Read that definition at least two more times before you read on. It's that important. And notice what comes up for you as you do. Does it feel scandalous? Illicit? Greedy? Impossible? Selfish? It's totally cool if you feel none of that and instead feel amazing! Whatever the case may be, just notice the feelings that come up. Those feelings are strong indicators of where you stand in your ability to receive.

If you feel intense feelings of negativity around receiving, I want to assure you that once you get started, receiving will be some of the best fun you've had in your life and on this journey. Being able to open yourself up to receive the things you desire in life is indeed vulnerable, but I assure you that it's worth the risk. Women in receiving mode are incredibly attractive and exude femininity. I bet you know women in your acquaintance now who are excellent at receiving. Maybe you've even judged them! *I know I did.* That judgment was simply jealousy. I wanted to be showered with love and my desires like those women allowed themselves to be. Instead of being jealous, join them!

I encourage you here to open your heart and mind up to the idea of Radical Receiving. In the past I have also referred to this as Ridiculous Receiving, but in our work here, I see it as radical because we are rediscovering what it means to receive within the larger context of reclaiming our feminine. When you get good at receiving, it will feel radical!

A great place to start is to review the definition of *receiving* I gave above daily. Write it down on something the size of a business card. Carry it around with you, and practice receiving the things listed in my definition. Receive gifts with a simple "thank you" rather than some senseless diatribe about how "they shouldn't have." Choose gratitude over shame when someone goes out of their way for you. Instead of tormenting yourself over the need to immediately reciprocate a kindness, let yourself revel in the joy of having received. I know from personal experience that the more I allowed myself to receive, the better my outlook on humanity was and the better "giver" I became. If you are the kind of person who expects a lugubrious display of gratitude when *you* give and falls into a bitter funk when *they* don't, I assure you that receiving is a place in the cosmology of your femininity that needs attention. The best receivers are truly the best givers.

Engaging Your Feminine *Daily*

When you are serious about improving anything, it's a daily thing. This is especially true with our intimate relationships. Your relationship with your feminine is exactly that: intimate. Your feminine is with you now and always has been. Decades of programming have made it harder to hear her. This is your chance to elevate her voice and have her walk alongside you in a more consistent and conscious way. Remember, your feminine is the part of you that feels. She's intuitive. She knows what she wants, even if it doesn't make sense to anyone else. She's creative. She's open to possibility. I am including these examples again because when you are rediscovering her, it's good to have loads of reminders. Under the tyranny of the masculine matrix, we get so stuck that it feels like we are learning an entirely new language when we are talking about the feminine. And, in some ways, we are.

What I would challenge you to do is check in with her daily. Make conversation with her a priority. The way I go about this is as follows: Immediately upon waking, I thank GUS for opening my eyes, giving me breath, giving me the gift of another day with those I love, and giving me the chance to make a difference in the lives of the women I serve. That all happens in the span of about fifteen seconds. I then call on my feminine to tell me what she needs. When it comes to the spiritual, creative, loving, nurturing, intuitive, abundant, and connected side of me, what does she need? If I don't hear anything immediately, I let her know that I trust she will nudge me throughout the day, and when I notice it, I will listen. I put no pressure on my feminine to blurt out an answer. She loves lingering in the question. The masculine is the part of you that demands an answer yesterday! Be open. This second part takes about fifteen seconds as well. That means that, in less than a minute, I have expressed gratitude to GUS and connected with my feminine. See how simple that is? We spend more time agonizing over how a connection like this "should" be rather than getting down to the business of actually making that connection.

My way is not the only way. I encourage you to take what I have shared here with you and play with it. Modify it. Make it your own. No candles, yoga poses, or ecstatic dance needed. If that stuff rings your bell, awesome. Just don't complicate it. The more complicated you make this, the more likely you will be sidetracked by excuses and perfectionism. Engage your feminine—daily.

The Feminine Loves Low Stress

The masculine matrix sold us on the idea that the more stressed you are, the more accomplished, important, productive, and, therefore, worthy you must be. In the United States, we've made stress a badge of honor. This is especially true for women. Whether in the workplace or at home, we got the message that you've got to martyr yourself to be great. Nonsense. It's just another means of masculinizing women to keep us weak, tired, and 100% out of our feminine power. Who says that we must be stress cases to do excellent work and to be great wives, mothers, and friends? In our culture, we make the stressed-out woman archetype the norm rather than questioning it. This is where you can line up with your feminine by deciding that the hardcore stress of your masculine is getting the boot.

I realize that the idea of *deciding* you aren't going to be a stress case might inspire a giant eye roll, but hear me out. Consistent and sustained stress is a choice. And because it's a choice, you can decide to stop buying into the lie that says it's your only option. You can make low stress your new normal through two critically important mechanisms: mindset and empowered choice. *Your feminine is going to love it—and it's awesome for your fertility.*

The Mindset of Feminine Responsibility

The mindset I am talking about here is a simple one, and it goes like this: *I am 100% responsible for how I feel.* You might read that and want to throw this book or the device you are reading it on out the window, but like it or not, it's true.

Chances are you have about a zillion *buts* going through your head right now, but you can't outrun or blame away this reality. We, as individuals, are responsible for attaching meaning to the things that show up and that *we create* in our lives. Objectively, your boss walking in on a Friday afternoon asking you to stay late to finish up some reports is simply your boss asking you to do something. All the meanings you attach to that event, such as "I always get picked on," "OMG, I'm going to lose my job if I say no," or "If I don't do this, everyone at work is going to hate me" are meanings of your own creation. You have no clue whether those things are currently true, but when you let those meanings hijack your thinking, you immediately render yourself powerless. The better approach mindset-wise, which your feminine will love because she's all about feeling and truth, is, "I am responsible for how I feel about this." This keeps you in the present rather than slipping into old stories from the past or going into future-tripping chaos about what "could happen" if you don't stay late.

Do you choose to be stressed about this or not? There's no right answer. It's simply your choice, and you are responsible for it.

When you put this into practice, you will see that the masculine matrix taught us to be stressed and insecure about everything, but we don't have to be. Bills will be paid, work will be done, babies will be birthed, and life will go on. We get to decide how we experience and feel each of those things. The feminine knows you have a choice. Let her guide you to making a better one than staying stuck in f*ck-with-your-fertility-level stress.

This leads us into the second mechanism of making low-stress normal: empowered choice. When you have a mindset based on the idea that you are 100% responsible for how you feel, you start making higher-quality choices. Empowered choice means you include your feminine in the conversation (Feminine First) to see what she has to say about what you're going to do. When we are stuck in our masculine, we are less discerning. *We just do.* We tell stories about what it means if we don't do the "right" masculine thing, we try to outwork our unworthiness, and we try to be all things to everyone. It's more masculine chasing and striving. The feminine checks in and asks if the choice you're about to make lines up with what you value and if what you are doing feels right. The feminine that fuels empowered choices is like an awesome traffic cop who tells us to speed up or slow down—from a place of love, not from a place of having to prove something. Empowered choice gives you a level of license and agency in your life that necessarily comes from looking at your life more holistically. There will be times when staying late at the office is exactly what your feminine guides you to do, but you can bet she will make sure you have a massage lined up the next day to help take the edge off. With your mindset right and empowered choice as your new normal, your feminine will be less "fried" and more free to come out and play.

It's an *And* Not *Or* Proposition

One of the most impactful moves you will make in reclaiming your feminine is to take a stand for *and*. My ladies hear me evangelizing about this all the time. The masculine matrix loves to create scenarios that aren't legit choices at all. "You can either stay home to raise your children, *or* you can do something meaningful with your life." See how that works? It's completely f*cked up. Who says staying home with your children isn't meaningful? Who says you can't get back into the workforce after your children are in school? Mama, that garbage is all made up. You get to have a family and a career if you wish! You can devote part of your life to your children and another part of your life to work. You give yourself permission to have *both*, a family and a career or any version of those things that feels right to you.

Here's something even crazier: *what if you choose not to work at all?* Let's say you choose to receive (there's that scary *r*-word) from your husband by letting him provide for you while you pursue hobbies, interests, and pregnancy. I raised that possibility in the last chapter, and I'm intentionally raising it again here, not because I'm trying to get you to do it, but because there's power in exploring the once verboten as a legitimate choice, even if it looks like a stretch from where you are today. You could give yourself permission to be a housewife (or a "domestic engineer," as my mom used to call it). How cool would that be? If your head is exploding at that suggestion, it might be because you love the idea but can't wrap your head around it yet. Can you imagine loving yourself and your husband or partner enough to allow yourself to be taken care of? Not because you are incapable of doing something yourself but because it feels good. Can you imagine *that*? It wouldn't be being oppressed, trapped in a kitchen, or damned to a life of laundry; it would just be what works for your growing family.

Let this idea roll around in your head. I realize that setup is not for everyone—for a multitude of reasons!—but the point was to get you thinking about the judgments you hold about it, the stories you've been told about receiving, what's "productive," how you "should" contribute to your family, and what decades in the masculine matrix have done to your perception. Sixty-plus years ago, staying home was a completely acceptable and lovely choice. Today it's virtually unheard of, and the first things people think when they come across a woman who doesn't work are "Concubine? Sister wife? Poor thing! Should I call for help?" If you feel any of that coming up, just smile. It's a sign your old judgments are triggered. Now you will be able to answer those judgments with, "I'm happy that she has chosen a life that's right for her!"

The masculine tries to bully us into either-or thinking. It's time to take a feminine approach to our lives by allowing and exercising the power of *and*.

Well-Curated Feminine Community

On your journey back to your feminine, you are going to need community—and I mean a *real* community of women who are cultivating their feminine too. I believe there's extraordinary power in surrounding yourself with like-minded women who are breaking out of the masculine stronghold they've been trapped in. When I was in the process of reclaiming my feminine, I couldn't be around women who were already super feminine. It's like learning to swim by jumping into a frozen lake. For me, it was too jarring. I needed to ease into it. Too much of the feminine too fast made me want to barf. I needed a chance to feel out what the feminine was for me—*then* I could go jumping in Femme Lake. If you feel the same, clearly, you aren't alone. There are thousands of other women reading this book now, too, who are sending out the accountability partner signal. I promise you will find them. Women reclaiming their feminine are everywhere. They are hilarious too. You will enjoy clumsily making your way back to the feminine together. You can cackle your way through it as you giddily discuss getting an intuitive hit from your feminine that said a nap at work was a good choice or how telling your mother-in-law to shove it just "felt true."

Once you get your bearings, then I encourage you to venture into deeper waters with older, wiser women who are deeply in their feminine. This was one of the power moves I made when reclaiming my own femininity. I sought out women outside of my family, sidestepping generational baggage about femininity, to be my guides. There was so much wisdom and experience they had to share with me. They were incredibly diverse in their expression of the feminine as well, which helped me gain a more well-rounded view of what mine could be. Some were feminine in countenance and manner, while others were more outwardly masculine but feminine in their approach to life. Yes, they were bosses at work, but when not at work, they slipped into their feminine masterfully and understood there was a place for each.

No Regrets, Just Pivot

Like a woman emerging from a dark cave into the full light of day, there may be part of you that wants to run back to the dark. When I say *to the dark*, I mean to the masculine matrix pattern of shame, guilt, and belief that there's only "one way." That may manifest in you beating yourself up for decisions you've made in the past while dominated by your masculine, against the advice of your feminine, aka your heart. Maybe what comes up for you is a career choice, a relationship you let go of, a pregnancy you terminated, things you've done or said in your current relationship, boundaries you've allowed to be porous, the years you've spent in exhaustion, or the life you haven't allowed yourself to live. Awakening has a funny way of dragging all those things up. You may not want to look at them because of the pain of regret they may bring up.

What if, instead of beating yourself up with regret, you just thanked past events for being a catalyst for your pivot to power, peace, and pregnancy? Talk about a break-free-from-the-masculine-matrix gangster move! Remember, you're reading this book so you can have your baby and live an amazing life. When the temptation to slip into regret pops up, shout, "Thanks for propelling my pivot!" No regrets, Mama. Just pivot.

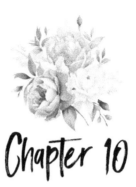

Chapter 10

Go Forth in Feminine —She's the Cure

I call what I've shared here with you the Feminine Fertility Cure because it is. If you are ever going to have a real chance at finally getting and staying pregnant, it won't be because of some treatment, diet, supplement, lotion, or potion you got your hands on. It will be because of who you allowed yourself to become. The woman who could see beyond her age, diagnosis, and statistics, beyond doubting loved ones and long-faced experts with lifeless proclamations, beyond her past, her failures, and her pain. The woman who allowed herself to experience love, excitement, joy, the present moment, trust, and faith...again. The version of you who is a gift to the children you've wept for. None of that comes from grinding, pushing, forcing, chasing, or blaming. It's found in the place you were taught not to look: the feminine.

Your feminine is what will lead you to make heart-centered, strategic, vision-based choices on this journey that lift you out of the fear, doubt, negativity, lack, and scarcity thinking that will sabotage your success. Your feminine is what guides you to live your life, work, relationships, and purpose differently so you can get out of the toxic stress trap that the data shows negatively impacts your fertility. Your feminine is what guides you to the mentors and healers that are instrumental in your success —*she led you to me, right?* Ignoring the curative power of your feminine is a rookie mistake. You're in the big leagues now, Mama. You can't unsee what I've shown you here. Your feminine is what has been missing from your journey, and your results show it. If you are serious about fertility success, you'll let her lead the way. She has this baby-making thing down. *It's pretty much what she's known for.*

What I've shared here is just a beginning. Like your fertility journey, the road back to your feminine is one of decision, trust, perseverance, and purpose. It's a daily decision and a commitment to living by truth in your life. The good news is that other women are waking up too. In the post-COVID era, women got a big taste of working from home and being more connected with their families.[1] Even though families were broken by the sixty-plus-years-long attack on the feminine, *the resurgence of the feminine will restore families.* No matter how hard the masculine matrix came at us, the funny thing is that we have still longed for babies and family. The matrix hated us for it, made us feel ashamed, unworthy, and even silly. But there was a deeper, innate GUS-inspired part of us that called us home to our feminine. Our job now is to let her reign.

Go forth in feminine, Mama. You get to have it all. A career, family, love, fulfillment, purpose, and joy. The difference here is that you will do it on your uniquely feminine terms. You are competing with no one. You are a woman, not a man. You get to live in your feminine glory, and there's nothing "lesser" about it.

---

1. Justin Palarino, Michael Burrows and Brian McKenzie, "Share of Remote Workers Tripled from 2019 to 2021, Most Were Women," United States Census Bureau, May 16, 2023, https://www.census.gov/library/stories/2023/05/women-majority-home-based-workers-during-pandemic.html.

Your unique expression of the feminine is your power. See value and purpose in the masculine and feminine that naturally live within you. Then appreciate the dance of the masculine and feminine in others. There's nothing the masculine matrix hates more than freedom, so find it in your Fearless Feminine.

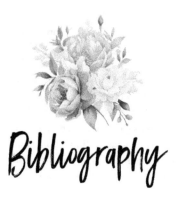

Bibliography

Adam, Jamela. "When Could Women Open a Bank Account?" Forbes Advisor. May 20, 2023. https://www.forbes.com/advisor/banking/when-could-women-open-a-bank-account/.

"Advance Report of Final Divorce Statistics, 1988." *Monthly Vital Statistics Report* 39, no. 12 (May 21, 1991). https://doi.org/10.18356/3023d8cd-en.

American Time Use Survey Summary - 2022 A01 Results. U.S. Bureau of Labor Statistics. June 22, 2023. https://www.bls.gov/news.release/atus.nro.htm.

Bump, Philip. "Baby Boomer." *Encyclopedia Britannica.* Last updated November 12, 2023. https://www.britannica.com/topic/baby-boomers.

"Betty Friedan." *Encyclopedia Britannica.* Last updated March 5, 2024. https://www.britannica.com/biography/Betty-Friedan.

Bhattarai, Abha. "Smaller Cakes, Shorter Dresses, Bigger Diamonds: The Pandemic Is Shaking Up the $73 Billion Wedding Industry." *Washington Post.* February 11, 2021. https://www.washingtonpost.com/road-to-recovery/2021/02/11/zoom-weddings-covid-diamond-rings/.

Bieber, Christy. "What Is a No Fault Divorce?" *Forbes.* July 26, 2023. https://www.forbes.com/advisor/legal/divorce/no-fault-divorce/.

Bouvier, Eden. "Elizabeth Holmes and The Case of Feminism." Write Like a Girl. Medium. March 21, 2022. https://medium.com/write-like-a-girl/elizabeth-holmes-and-the-case-of-feminism-a-particularly-interesting-case-study-e4ff54d4b489.

"The Brady Bunch." *Encyclopedia Britannica.* November 17, 2023. https://www.britannica.com/topic/The-Brady-Bunch.

Brody, Debra J., and Qiuping Gu. "Antidepressant Use Among Adults: United States, 2015-2018." Centers for Disease Control and Prevention. September 2020. https://www.cdc.gov/nchs/products/databriefs/db377.htm.

Castleman, Michael. "This Is Why Many Women Watch Porn." Psychology Today. June 1, 2020. https://www.psychologytoday.com/us/blog/all-about-sex/202006/is-why-many-women-watch-porn.

"Census Bureau Reports 'Delayer Boom' as More Educated Women Have Children Later." United States Census Bureau. May 9, 2011. https://www.census.gov/newsroom/releases/archives/fertility/cb11-83.html.

"Changes in Men's and Women's Labor Force Participation Rates." U.S. Bureau of Labor Statistics. January 10, 2007. https://www.bls.gov/opub/ted/2007/jan/wk2/art03.htm.

Cohn, D'Vera, Gretchen Livingston, and Wendy Wang. "After Decades of Decline, A Rise in Stay-at Home Mothers." Pew Research Center. April 8, 2014. https://www.pewresearch.org/social-trends/2014/04/08/after-decades-of-decline-a-rise-in-stay-at-home-mothers/.

Dresden, Hilton. "Hollywood Flashback: 'Alice' Served Up a Hit for CBS in 1976." *Hollywood Reporter*. December 16, 2022. https://www.hollywoodreporter.com/tv/tv-news/hollywood-flashback-alice-cbs-1235283325/.

Featherstone, Liza. "Is It Just Us, or Is Girl-Boss Feminism Waning?" *Jacobin*. September 26, 2023. https://jacobin.com/2023/09/liberal-feminism-girl-boss-decline-hillary-clinton-one-percent.

Fertility Clinics in the US - Market Size (2004–2029). IBISWorld Industry Reports. November 15, 2023. https://www.ibisworld.com/industry-statistics/market-size/fertility-clinics-united-states/.

"Figure MS-1b: Women's Marital Status in Decennial Censuses, 1950 to 1990 and Current Population Survey Annual Social and Economic Supplements, 1993 to 2023." In *Decennial Censuses, 1950 to 1990, and Current Population Survey, Annual Social and Economic Supplements, 1993 to 2023*. U.S. Census Bureau. Last updated November 21, 2023. https://www.census.gov/content/dam/Census/library/visualizations/time-series/demo/families-and-households/ms-1b.pdf.

Fileva, Iskra. "Is Marriage a Bad Deal for Women?" Psychology Today. May 16, 2021. https://www.psychologytoday.com/us/blog/the-philosophers-diaries/202105/is-marriage-a-bad-deal-for-women.

Gill, Martha. " 'Girlboss' Used to Suggest a Kind of Role Model. How Did it Become a Sexist Putdown?" *Guardian* (US). August 21, 2022. https://www.theguardian.com/commentisfree/2022/aug/21/girlboss-used-to-suggest-role-model-sexist-putdown.

Golden, Claudia, Lawrence F. Katz, and Ilyana Kuziemko. "The Homecoming of American College Women: The Reversal of the College Gender Gap."

Journal of Economic Perspectives 20, no. 4 (2006): 133–56. https://doi.org/10.1257/jep.20.4.133.

Hamilton, B. E., et al. "Natality Trends in the United States, 1909–2018." National Center for Health Statistics. Last updated July 12, 2018. https://www.cdc.gov/nchs/data-visualization/natality-trends/index.htm.

Hershkowitz, Donna S., and Drew R. Liebert. *The Direction of Divorce Reform in California: From Fault to No-Fault...and Back Again?* Sacramento, CA: Assembly Judiciary Committee. California State Legislature. 1997. https://ajud.assembly.ca.gov/sites/ajud.assembly.ca.gov/files/reports/1197%20divorcereform97.pdf.

Hymowitz, Kay S. "The Indispensable Institution." *City Journal.* September 15, 2023. https://www.city-journal.org/article/review-of-the-two-parent-privilege-by-melissa-kearney.

"Infertility FAQs." Centers for Disease Control and Prevention. Last updated April 26, 2023. https://www.cdc.gov/reproductivehealth/infertility/index.htm.

Imrie, Rachel, Srirupa Ghosh, Nitish Narvekar, Kugajeevan Vigneswaran, Yanzhong Wang, and Mike Savvas. "Socioeconomic Status and Fertility Treatment Outcomes in High-Income Countries: A Review of the Current Literature." *Human Fertility* 26, no. 1 (2023): 27–37. https://doi.org/10.1080/14647273.2021.1957503.

Joannides, Paul. "What Women Want in a Man." Psychology Today. November 1, 2023. https://www.psychologytoday.com/us/blog/as-you-like-it/202310/what-women-want-in-a-man/.

Kearney, Melissa, Phillip Levine, and Luke Pardue. "The Mystery of the Declining U.S. Birth Rate." EconoFact. February 15, 2022. https://econofact.org/the-mystery-of-the-declining-u-s-birth-rate.

Kearney, Melissa S., Phillip B. Levine, and Luke Pardue. "The Puzzle of Falling US Birth Rates since the Great Recession." *Journal of Economic Perspectives* 36, no. 1 (Winter 2022): 151–76. https://doi.org/10.1257/jep.36.1.151.

Kearney, Melissa S., Phillip B. Levine, and Luke Pardue. *The Two-Parent Privilege: How Americans Stopped Getting Married and Started Falling Behind.* Chicago, IL: University of Chicago Press, 2023.

Keller, Jon. "Keller @ Large: The Brady Bunch Changed How Americans Viewed Women." CBS News. July 12, 2011. https://www.cbsnews.com/boston/news/keller-large-the-brady-bunch-changed-how-americans-viewed-women/.

Knapton, Sarah. "Bright Flash of Light Marks Incredible Moment Life Begins When Sperm Meets Egg." *Telegraph* (UK). April 26, 2016. https://www.telegraph.co.uk/science/2016/04/26/bright-flash-of-light-marks-incredible-moment-life-begins-when-s/.

Leiva, Ludmila. "Rejected for Being 'Too Successful': Career-Driven Women

Say It's Ruining Their Chances of Finding Love." Refinery29. September 25, 2018. https://www.refinery29.com/en-us/successful-women-dating-men.

Lell, Shannon. "I'm a Feminist Who's Attracted to 'Manly Men.' " *Washington Post.* September 13, 2016. https://www.washingtonpost.com/news/soloish/wp/2016/09/13/im-a-feminist-whos-attracted-to-manly-men/.

Livingston, Gretchen. "For Most Highly Educated Women, Motherhood Doesn't Start Until the 30s." Pew Research Center. January 15, 2015. https://www.pewresearch.org/short-reads/2015/01/15/for-most-highly-educated-women-motherhood-doesnt-start-until-the-30s/.

Livingston, Gretchen. "They're Waiting Longer, but U.S. Women Today More Likely to Have Children than a Decade Ago." Pew Research Center. January 18, 2018. https://www.pewresearch.org/social-trends/2018/01/18/theyre-waiting-longer-but-u-s-women-today-more-likely-to-have-children-than-a-decade-ago/.

Luu, Zoe. "The Irony of #Girlboss Feminism." The Women's Network. May 26, 2022. https://www.thewomens.network/blog/the-irony-of-girlboss-feminism.

Lynch, Courtney Denning-Johnson, Rajeshwari Sundaram, José M. Maisog, A.M. Sweeney, and Germaine M. Buck Louis. "Preconception Stress Increases the Risk of Infertility: Results from a Couple-Based Prospective Cohort Study—The LIFE Study." *Human Reproduction* 29, no. 5 (2014): 1067–75. https://doi.org/10.1093/humrep/deu032.

Malone, Joe. "What's Happening in Male vs. Female Brains During Sex?" Natural Womanhood. February 17, 2023. https://naturalwomanhood.org/what-happens-in-mens-vs-women-brains-during-sex/.

Marcinkowska, Urszula M., Markus J. Rantala, Anthony J. Lee, Mikhail V. Kozlov, Toivo Aavik, Huajian Cai, Jorge Contreras-Garduño, Oana A. David, Gwenaël Kaminski, Norman P. Li, Ike E. Onyishi, Keshav Prasai, Farid Pazhoohi, Pavol Prokop, Sandra L. Rosales Cardozo, Nicolle Sydney, Hirokazu Taniguchi, Indrikis Krams, and Barnaby J. W. Dixson."Women's Preferences for Men's Facial Masculinity Are Strongest Under Favorable Ecological Conditions." *Scientific Reports* 9, no. 1 (2019): 3387. https://doi.org/10.1038/s41598-019-39350-8.

"The Mary Tyler Moore Show." *Encyclopedia Britannica.* Last updated January 25, 2024. https://www.britannica.com/topic/The-Mary-Tyler-Moore-Show.

McCammon, Sarah. "How the Approval of the Birth Control Pill 60 Years Ago Helped Change Lives." Houston Public Media. May 9, 2020. https://www.houstonpublicmedia.org/npr/2020/05/09/852807455/how-the-approval-of-the-birth-control-pill-60-years-ago-helped-change-lives/.

McKenna, Amy. "Generation X." *Encyclopedia Britannica.* March 1, 2024. https://www.britannica.com/topic/Generation-X.

Mohan, Pavithra. "This Pandemic Isn't the First Time Women Have Left the Workforce in Droves." *Fast Company.* March 29, 2021. https://www.fastcom

pany.com/90617765/this-pandemic-isnt-the-first-time-women-have-left-the-workforce-in-droves.

Palarino, Justin, Michael Burrows, and Brian McKenzie. "Share of Remote Workers Tripled from 2019 to 2021; Most Were Women." United States Census Bureau. May 16, 2023. https://www.census.gov/library/stories/2023/05/women-majority-home-based-workers-during-pandemic.html.

Paul, Kari. "Elizabeth Holmes Objects to $250 Monthly Payments to Theranos Victims." *Guardian* (US), June 14, 2023. https://www.theguardian.com/us-news/2023/jun/14/elizabeth-holmes-theranos-victims-repayment-objection.

Peltzman, Sam. "The Socio-Political Demography of Happiness." Working Paper, George J. Stigler Center for the Study of the Economy & the State. https://dx.doi.org/10.2139/ssrn.4508123.

"The Pill and the Sexual Revolution." PBS. Accessed April 11, 2024. https://www.pbs.org/wgbh/americanexperience/features/pill-and-sexual-revolution/.

Piper, Kelsey. "A New Book Says Married Women Are Miserable. Don't Believe It." Vox. June 4, 2019. https://www.vox.com/future-perfect/2019/6/4/18650969/married-women-miserable-fake-paul-dolan-happiness.

Rasmussen, Tom. "I Couldn't Help But Wonder...Should Women Have Sex Like Men?" *Vogue.* November 3, 2022. https://www.vogue.com/article/women-sex-like-men.

"Roe v. Wade Is Decided, January 22, 1973." History.com. Accessed April 11, 2024. https://www.history.com/this-day-in-history/roe-v-wade.

Rooney, Kristin L., and Alice D. Domar. "The Relationship between Stress and Infertility." *Dialogues in Clinical Neuroscience* 20, no. 1 (2018), 41–47. https://doi.org/10.31887/DCNS.2018.20.1/klrooney.

Rosen, Ruth. "Who Said 'We Could Have It All'?" openDemocracy. August 2, 2012. https://www.opendemocracy.net/en/5050/who-said-we-could-have-it-all/.

Stanton, Glenn T. "The Pill: Did It Cause the Sexual Revolution?" Focus on the Family. July 6, 2010. https://www.focusonthefamily.com/marriage/the-pill-did-it-cause-the-sexual-revolution/.

Stevenson, Betsey, and Justin Wolfers. "The Paradox of Declining Female Happiness." Working Paper, National Bureau of Economic Research, 2009. https://www.nber.org/papers/w14969.

Thomas, Susan Gregory. "All Apologies: Thank You for the 'Sorry.' " HuffPost. August 23, 2011. https://www.huffpost.com/entry/all-apologies-thank-you-f_b_931718.

Toossi, Mitra, and Teresa L. Morisi. "Women in the Workforce Before, During, and After the Great Recession: Spotlight on Statistics." U.S. Bureau of Labor Statistics. July 2017. https://www.bls.gov/spotlight/2017/women-in-the-workforce-before-during-and-after-the-great-recession/home.htm.

"U.S. Fertility Rate 1950–2023." MacroTrends. Accessed November 26, 2023. https://www.macrotrends.net/countries/USA/united-states/fertility-rate.

Venker, Suzanne. "Why Super-Successful Women Struggle in Love." *Washington Examiner.* October 9, 2019. https://www.washingtonexaminer.com/opinion/1823575/why-super-successful-women-struggle-in-love/.

"What Happens to Your Body During the Fight-or-Flight Response?" Cleveland Clinic. December 8, 2019. https://health.clevelandclinic.org/what-happens-to-your-body-during-the-fight-or-flight-response

White, Ruth C. "No Strings Attached Sex (NSA): Can Women Really Do It?" Psychology Today. November 20, 2011. https://www.psychologytoday.com/us/blog/culture-in-mind/201111/no-strings-attached-sex-nsa-can-women-really-do-it.

Wilcox, Brad, and Wendy Wang. "The Married-Mom Advantage." *Atlantic,* December 27, 2022. https://www.theatlantic.com/ideas/archive/2022/12/motherhood-marriage-pandemic-covid-children/672563/.

Woods, Amy. "Fashion Empowers Ambition: The Evolution of Women's Workwear." The Women's Network. Accessed April 11, 2024. https://www.thewomens.network/blog/fashion-empowers-ambition-the-evolution-of-womens-workwear.

"Women in the Workforce: 1970s - A Decade of Change." HR & PEO Services for Small Business. October 20, 2022. https://www.propelhr.com/blog/women-in-the-workforce-1970s-a-decade-of-change-for-women.

Yellen, Janet L. "The History of Women's Work and Wages and How it Has Created Success for Us All." Brookings. May 2020. https://www.brookings.edu/articles/the-history-of-womens-work-and-wages-and-how-it-has-created-success-for-us-all/.

"Yinyang." *Encyclopedia Britannica.* Last modified December 4, 2023. https://www.britannica.com/topic/yinyang.

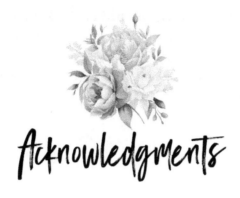

Acknowledgments

To my two main men, Brandon and Asher. Thank you for putting up with me on the nights when I worked way too late, missed dinner, or got a little grouchy. Making space for my work and my process was a sacrifice and an incredible act of love. I love how you love me.

To my ladies around the world. Thank you for your trust. You and your babies are the lights of my professional life. I hope you never forget how powerful you are.

To my editor, Yna. Your loving and hilarious genius always brings out the best in me. Thank you for helping me take my vision to the next level and guiding me out of the rabbit holes when needed. I can't wait to see what we create next.

To Shreddy, Auggie, Rambo, Shelby, and Vincent. Thank you for keeping me company as I wrote late into the night when Dad and Asher were asleep. Interestingly enough, you always helped me find the right words.

To GUS. Thank you for my fertility journey. Even in the

darkest moments, I knew you had my back. Your love ignited the courage in me to turn my pain into purpose. You always put the right books, teachers, mentors, and experiences in my life to keep me moving forward. You never fail to show me my truest *hell yes*.

About The Author

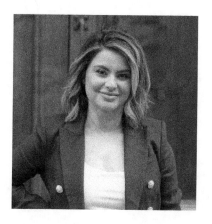

Rosanne Austin, JD, three-time bestselling author and creator of the Fearlessly Fertile Method, is a former state prosecutor turned Fertility Fairy Godmother. She is the fertility mentor physicians trust and women around the world turn to when they are committed to mama-making success. Rosanne overcame her own seven-year struggle with fertility and had her son naturally at almost forty-four, when medicine had given up on her. She is committed to helping women get and stay pregnant. With her books, podcast, online courses, and retreats, Rosanne helps her clients become the moms they were meant to be. She resides in The Woodlands, Texas, with her husband, son, two chihuahuas, one rottweiler, and two formerly feral cats. When she's not writing, mentoring, or chasing her son around, she loves traveling, deep conversation, high tea, and Jane Austen movie marathons.

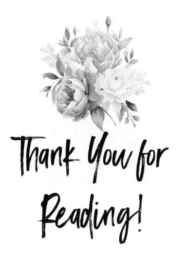

Thank You for Reading!

Want a mantra that will help you stay focused on your new relationship with your fertility superpower?

I've put the empowering nine-word mantra that I lived by during my own fertility journey on a phone wallpaper, *just for you!*

To thank you for finishing my book, I want to share the mantra that kept me feeling confident and free. My Miracle Mamas around the world use it too!

This gorgeous wallpaper for your device will keep you focused on the *nine* words that will steady you in any situation that shows up on your journey.

And saying this mantra feels so good you'll want to *SHOUT IT!*

Save it to your phone or print it and tuck it into your back pocket so it's there to keep you living your pregnancy with ease and joy.

Get your FREE Fearless Feminine mantra wallpaper *now!*

Scan the QR code or go to https://www.frommaybetobaby.com/ ffc-gift-2.